MORE 4U!

the _____ n

This Clinics series is available online.

**ere's what
u get:**

- Full text of EVERY issue from 2002 to NOW
- Figures, tables, drawings, references and more
- Searchable: find what you need fast

  Search [All Clinics ▼] for [   ] [GO]

- Linked to MEDLINE and Elsevier journals
- E-alerts

**DIVIDUAL
BSCRIBERS**

LOG ON TODAY. IT'S FAST AND EASY.

ck **Register**
d follow
structions

u'll need your
count number

Your subscriber
account number
is on your mailing
label

> This is your copy of:
> THE CLINICS OF NORTH AMERICA
> CXXX   **2296532-2**   2   Mar 05
>
> J.H. DOE, MD
> 531 MAIN STREET
> CENTER CITY, NY 10001-001

BOUGHT A SINGLE ISSUE? Sorry, you won't be able
to access full text online. Please subscribe today to get
complete content by contacting customer service at
800 645 2452 (US and Canada) or 407 345 4000 (outside
US and Canada) or via email at elsols@elsevier.com.

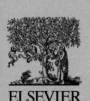

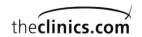

OBSTETRICS AND GYNECOLOGY CLINICS

OF NORTH AMERICA

Preterm Labor: Prediction and Treatment

GUEST EDITOR
John C. Morrison, MD

September 2005 • Volume 32 • Number 3

SAUNDERS

An Imprint of Elsevier, Inc.
PHILADELPHIA   LONDON   TORONTO   MONTREAL   SYDNEY   TOKYO

W.B. SAUNDERS COMPANY
A Division of Elsevier Inc.

Elsevier, Inc. • 1600 John F. Kennedy Blvd. • Suite 1800 • Philadelphia, PA 19103-2899

http://www.theclinics.com

OBSTETRICS AND GYNECOLOGY
CLINICS OF NORTH AMERICA
September 2005
Editor: Carin Davis

Volume 32, Number 3
ISSN 0889-8545
ISBN 1-4160-2743-2

The ideas and opinions expressed in *Obstetrics and Gynecology Clinics of North America* do not necessarily reflect those of the Publisher. The Publisher does not assume any responsibility for any injury and/or damage to persons or property arising out of or related to any use of the material contained in this periodical. The reader is advised to check the appropriate medical literature and the product information currently provided by the manufacturer of each drug to be administered to verify the dosage, the method and duration of administration, or contraindications. It is the responsibility of the treating physician or other health care professional, relying on independent experience and knowledge of the patient, to determine drug dosages and the best treatment for the patient. Mention of any product in this issue should not be construed as endorsement by the contributors, editors, or the Publisher of the product or manufacturers' claims.

Obstetrics and Gynecology Clinics of North America (ISSN 0889-8545) is published quarterly by Elsevier Inc. Corporate and editorial offices: Elsevier, Inc., 1600 John F. Kennedy Blvd., Suite 1800, Philadelphia, PA 19103-2899. Accounting and circulation offices: 6277 Sea Harbor Drive, Orlando, FL 32887-4800. Periodicals postage paid at Orlando, FL 32862, and additional mailing offices. Subscription prices are $175.00 per year for US individuals, $288.00 per year for US institutions, $88.00 per year for US students and residents, $207.00 per year for Canadian individuals, $350.00 per year for Canadian institutions, $235.00 per year for international individuals, $350.00 per year for international institutions and $118.00 per year for Canadian and foreign students/residents. To receive student/resident rate, orders must be accompanied by name of affiliated institution, date of term, and the signature of program/residency coordinator on institution letterhead. Orders will be billed at individual rate until proof of status is received. Foreign air speed delivery is included in all Clinics subscription prices. All prices are subject to change without notice. POSTMASTER: Send address changes to *Obstetrics and Gynecology Clinics of North America*, W.B. Saunders Company, Periodicals Fulfillment, Orlando, FL 32887-4800. **Customer Service: 1-800-654-2452 (US). From outside of the US, call 1-407-345-4000.**

Obstetrics and Gynecology Clinics of North America is also published in Spanish by Mc Graw-Hill Interamericana Editores S.A., P.O. Box 5-237, 06500, Mexico; in Portuguese by Reichmann and Affonso Editores, Rio de Janeiro, Brazil; and in Greek by Paschalidis Medical Publications, Athens, Greece.

Obstetrics and Gynecology Clinics of North America is covered in *Index Medicus, Excerpta Medica, Current Concepts/Clinical Medicine, Science Citation Index, BIOSIS, CINAHL, and ISI/BIOMED.*

Printed in the United States of America.

GOAL STATEMENT

The goal of *Obstetrics and Gynecology Clinics of North America* is to keep practicing physicians up to date with current clinical practice in OB/GYN by providing timely articles reviewing the state of the art in patient care.

ACCREDITATION

The *Obstetrics and Gynecology Clinics of North America* is planned and implemented in accordance with the Essential Areas and Policies of the Accreditation Council for Continuing Medical Education (ACCME) through the joint sponsorship of the University of Virginia School of Medicine and Elsevier. The University of Virginia School of Medicine is accredited by the ACCME to provide continuing medical education for physicians.

The University of Virginia School of Medicine designates this educational activity for a maximum of 60 category 1 credits per year, 15 category 1 credits per issue, toward the AMA Physician's Recognition Award. Each physician should claim only those credits that he/she actually spent in the activity.

The American Medical Association has determined that physicians not licensed in the US who participate in this CME activity are eligible for AMA PRA category 1 credit.

Category 1 credit can be earned by reading the text material, taking the CME examination online at http://www.theclinics.com/home/cme, and completing the evaluation. After taking the test, you will be required to review any and all incorrect answers. Following completion of the test and evaluation, your credit will be awarded and you may print your certificate.

FACULTY DISCLOSURE

Faculty Disclosure

As a provider accredited by the Accreditation Council for Continuing Medical Education (ACCME), the Office of Continuing Medical Education of the University of Virginia School of Medicine must ensure balance, independence, objectivity, and scientific rigor in all its individually sponsored or jointly sponsored educational activities. All authors/editors participating in a sponsored activity are expected to disclose to the readers any significant financial interest or other relationship (1) with the manufacturer(s) of any commercial product(s) and/or provider(s) of commercial services discussed in an educational presentation and (2) with any commercial supporters of the activity (significant financial interest or other relationship can include such things as grants or research support, employee, consultant, stock holder, member of speakers bureau, etc.) The intent of this disclosure is not to prevent authors/editors with a significant financial or other relationship from writing an article, but rather to provide readers with information on which they can make their own judgments. It remains for the readers to determine whether the author's/editor's interest or relationships may influence the article with regard to exposition or conclusion.

The authors/editors listed below have identified no professional or financial affiliations related to their article:

Adrienne Z. Ables, PharmD; George Bega, MD; Michele Berghella, MD; Vincenzo Berghella, MD; Sunett P. Chauhan, MD; Carin Davis, Acquisitions Editor; Ronald S. Gibbs, MD; Pamela Gill Lam, MSN, RN; Laura L. Klein, MD; Fung Lam, MD; David F. Lewis, MD, MBA; George C. Lu, MD; Brian M. Mercer, MD; John C. Morrison, MD; Amen Ness, MD; Roger B. Newman, MD; William E. Roberts, MD; Christopher J. Robinson, MD; Ana Maria Romero, MD; Orion A. Rust, MD; Stephen T. Vermillion, MD; and, John D. Yeast, MD, MSPH.

The author listed below has identified the following professional or financial affiliation related to the article:
John P. Elliot, MD is on the speakers' bureau for Matria Healthcare.

Disclosure of discussion of non-FDA approved uses for pharmaceutical products and/or medical devices: The University of Virginia School of Medicine, as an ACCME provider, requires that all authors/editors identify and disclose any "off label" uses for pharmaceutical products and/or for medical devices. The University of Virginia School of Medicine recommends that each reader fully review all the available data on new products or procedures prior to instituting them with patients.

All authors/editors who provided disclosures have indicated that they will not be discussing off-label uses except:
Adrienne Z. Ables, PharmD, Sunett P. Chauhan, MD and Ana Maria Romero, MD will discuss the use of calcium channel blockers for preterm labor; all are off-label. Specifically, Nifedipine is referred to in the article.
Fung Lam, MD and Pamela Gill Lam, MSN, RN discuss intravenous magnesium sulfate tocolysis, orla terbutaline tocolysis, and sucutaneous terbutaline pump tocolysis.
David F. Lewis, MD, MBA discussed the use of magesium sulfate, terbutaline, indomethocin, and procardia as a tocolytic, to stop preterm labor.
Brian M. Mercer, MD will discuss the use of antibiotic therapy during conservative management of PROM.
William E. Roberts, MD and Orion A. Rust, MD discuss the use of indometacin for anti-inflammatory and uterine tocolytic effects.
Christopher J. Robinson, MD discussed the use of celocoxib as an investigational agent in tocolytic therapy for preterm labor.

TO ENROLL

To enroll in the *Obstetrics and Gynecology Clinics of North America* Continuing Medical Education program, call customer service at 1-800-654-2452 or visit us online at www.theclinics.com/home/cme. The CME program is available to subscribers for an additional fee of $99.95.

GUEST EDITOR

JOHN C. MORRISON, MD, Professor, Department of Obstetrics, Gynecology, and Pediatrics, University of Mississippi Medical Center, Jackson, Mississippi

CONTRIBUTORS

ADRIENNE Z. ABLES, PharmD, Associate Professor of Family Medicine, Spartanburg Family Medicine Residency Program, Spartanburg, South Carolina

GEORGE BEGA, MD, Research Assistant and Professor, Division of Maternal-Fetal Medicine, Department of Obstetrics and Gynecology, Jefferson Medical College of Thomas Jefferson University, Philadelphia, Pennsylvania

MICHELE BERGHELLA, MD, Department of Obstetrics and Gynecology, Ospedale 'SS Trinita,' Pescara, Italy

VINCENZO BERGHELLA, MD, Associate Professor and Director, Division of Maternal-Fetal Medicine; Director, Maternal-Fetal Medicine Fellowship Program, Department of Obstetrics and Gynecology, Jefferson Medical College of Thomas Jefferson University, Philadelphia, Pennsylvania

SUNEET P. CHAUHAN, MD, Department of Medical Education and Maternal-Fetal Medicine, Spartanburg Regional Medical Center, Spartanburg, South Carolina

JOHN P. ELLIOTT, MD, Partner, Phoenix Perinatal Associates, a Division of Obstetrix Medical Group of Phoenix; Director, Division of Maternal-Fetal Medicine, Banner Good Samaritan Medical Center, Phoenix, Arizona

RONALD S. GIBBS, MD, Professor and Chair, Department of Obstetrics and Gynecology, University of Colorado Health Sciences Center, Denver, Colorado

PAMELA GILL, RN, MSN, Department of Obstetrics and Gynecology, California Pacific Medical Center, San Francisco, California

LAURA L. KLEIN, MD, Fellow, Maternal Fetal Medicine, Department of Obstetrics and Gynecology, University of Colorado Health Sciences Center, Denver, Colorado

FUNG LAM, MD, Clinical Professor, Department of Obstetrics, Gynecology and Reproductive Sciences, University of California, San Francisco; California Pacific Medical Center, San Francisco, California

DAVID F. LEWIS, MD, Professor and Chairman, Department of Obstetrics and Gynecology, Louisiana State University Health Sciences Center, Shreveport, Louisiana

GEORGE LU, MD, Assistant Professor of Obstetrics and Gynecology, University of Missouri-Kansas City; Obstetrix Medical Group of Kansas and Missouri, Kansas City, Missouri

BRIAN M. MERCER, MD, FACOG, Professor of Reproductive Biology, Vice-Chair of Obstetrics and Gynecology, Director of Maternal-Fetal Medicine, Case Western Reserve University, MetroHealth Medical Center, Cleveland, Ohio

AMEN NESS, MD, Fellow, Division of Maternal-Fetal Medicine, Department of Obstetrics and Gynecology, Jefferson Medical College of Thomas Jefferson University, Philadelphia, Pennsylvania

ROGER B. NEWMAN, MD, Director, Division of Maternal Fetal Medicine, Vice-Chairman and Professor, Department of Obstetrics and Gynecology, Medical University of South Carolina, Charleston, South Carolina

WILLIAM E. ROBERTS, MD, Division of Maternal Fetal Medicine, Department of Obstetrics and Gynecology, Lehigh Valley Hospital, Allentown, Pennsylvania

CHRISTOPHER J. ROBINSON, MD, Clinical Instructor, Division of Maternal Fetal Medicine, Department of Obstetrics and Gynecology, Medical University of South Carolina, Charleston, South Carolina

ANA MARIA ROMERO, MD, Family Medicine Resident, Spartanburg Family Medicine Residency Program, Spartanburg, South Carolina

ORION A. RUST, MD, Division of Maternal Fetal Medicine, Department of Obstetrics and Gynecology, Lehigh Valley Hospital, Allentown, Pennsylvania

STEPHEN T. VERMILLION, MD, Associate Professor, Division of Maternal Fetal Medicine, Department of Obstetrics and Gynecology, Medical University of South Carolina, Charleston, South Carolina

JOHN D. YEAST, MD, MSPH, Professor of Obstetrics and Gynecology, University of Missouri-Kansas City; Director of Medical Affairs, Saint Luke's Hospital of Kansas City, Kansas City, Missouri

CONTENTS

> Few approaches to preterm birth prevention have been as thoroughly studied yet as enigmatic as uterine contraction assessment. Despite multiple randomized clinical trials (level 1 evidence), the effectiveness of home uterine contraction assessment as an adjunct to the clinical management of women at risk for preterm birth remains controversial. This article reviews these trials with particular attention to study design and patient inclusion criteria. The data are absolutely clear that home uterine contraction monitoring with or without frequent perinatal nursing contact can reduce the risk of preterm birth and improve perinatal outcomes and that both are independently superior to standard preterm birth prevention education and care.

> Premature labor and subsequent premature delivery is the major cause of perinatal death in the world. Numerous risk factors identify patients at jeopardy for preterm labor, but with poor sensitivity. Several biologic and biochemical markers have been recently studied that may allow early identification of patients at risk of preterm delivery. Although two markers have received Food and Drug Administration approval, a number of other tests also may ultimately prove useful.

ELSEVIER
SAUNDERS

Obstet Gynecol Clin N Am
32 (2005) xiii–xiv

OBSTETRICS AND
GYNECOLOGY
CLINICS
OF NORTH AMERICA

Preface

Preterm Labor: Prediction and Treatment

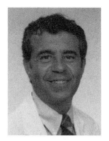

John C. Morrison, MD
Guest Editor

Preterm labor and the attendant complication of preterm delivery assure its position as the most common, costly, and catastrophic complication of pregnancy. Although preterm birth rates have risen during the past two decades, the majority of this increase has been due to the aggressive management of medical/surgical disorders requiring early delivery, assisted reproductive technologies resulting in a large number of higher-order multifetal gestations, and physician-allowed deliveries near term (>32.34 weeks). On the other hand, preterm births arising from labor before 37 weeks and spontaneous rupture of the membranes due to preterm labor have actually decreased as a result of enhanced use of preterm prediction techniques and aggressive, individualized treatment of preterm labor when it occurs. Progress has also been made toward understanding the multifactorial etiology of preterm labor and comprehensive management efforts toward preventing preterm birth have also made great contributions. These efforts have resulted in fewer preterm births, and overall better outcomes for mothers, babies, and families.

In this issue of the *Obstetrics and Gynecology Clinics of North America*, some of the best-known clinicians offer their thoughts in the specific areas of prediction techniques for an early diagnosis of preterm labor and individualized treatment in women who develop this problem. I really believe that this work will enable clinicians to practically manage women who are at risk for preterm birth and those who develop preterm labor. I also wish to thank Rosie McMillon, my

doi:10.1016/j.ogc.2005.07.001   *obgyn.theclinics.com*

secretary at the University of Mississippi Medical Center, and Carin Davis, Senior Editor at Elsevier, both of whom have prodded this work toward fruition.

John C. Morrison, MD
Department of Obstetrics, Gynecology and Pediatrics
University of Mississippi Medical Center
2500 North State Street
Jackson, MS 39216, USA
E-mail address: jmorrison@ob-gyn.umsmed.edu

ELSEVIER
SAUNDERS

Obstet Gynecol Clin N Am
32 (2005) 341–367

OBSTETRICS AND
GYNECOLOGY
CLINICS
OF NORTH AMERICA

Uterine Contraction Assessment

Roger B. Newman, MD

*Division of Maternal Fetal Medicine, Department of Obstetrics and Gynecology,
Medical University of South Carolina, 96 Jonathan Lucas Street, Charleston, SC 29425, USA*

The last quarter century has been marked by a persistent rise in the rate of preterm birth in the United States. This rising rate of preterm birth represents the failure of modern obstetrics to understand the complexity of the phenomena and to develop effective preterm birth prevention interventions. Of the many approaches to preterm birth prevention that have been investigated, no single intervention has been as thoroughly studied or as enigmatic as uterine contraction assessment. Uterine contraction assessment, or home uterine activity monitoring (HUAM) as it is more commonly known, has been subjected to some of the most rigorous testing ever applied to an obstetric intervention. Unfortunately, the effectiveness of uterine contraction assessment as an adjunct to the clinical management of women at risk for preterm birth became obscured by the overuse for indications with reduced risk for early delivery. Both academic and community obstetricians and gynecologists became polarized in their views regarding HUAM. As a result, much of the published literature regarding this intervention, including numerous randomized clinical trials, has been overstated or underconsidered depending on the clinician's pre-existing bias or clinical impression.

The frustrating thing about evidence-based medicine is that the results are not always consistent and the evidence frequently generates more questions than it answers. Why is it that in some investigations HUAM or uterine activity surveillance has been clearly beneficial for women at high risk of preterm delivery, whereas in others this approach seems to lack any significant benefit? Evidence-based medicine is only useful when one pays as much attention to the methodology as to the results. This article explores what has been learned about uterine contraction assessment when used as part of a comprehensive management program for women at risk for preterm delivery. This intervention is considered

E-mail address: newmanr@musc.edu

doi:10.1016/j.ogc.2005.04.005   *obgyn.theclinics.com*

in terms of its evolution through the 1980s and 1990s. The data for and against uterine activity assessment are outlined with particular attention to study design and patient inclusion criteria. With an appreciation of the methodology involved in each of these studies addressing uterine activity monitoring, a surprisingly clear picture emerges from what many people believe to be highly contradictory level 1 evidence.

Normal uterine contractility

Before specifically addressing the clinical use of uterine contraction assessment it is wise to consider the general topic of antepartum uterine contractility and its relationship to prematurity. In 1950, Alvarez and Caldeyro-Barcia [1] reported simply that "the uterus never sleeps." In pioneering studies they placed transabdominal intramyometrial pressure manometers to sequentially measure uterine pressures from early pregnancy through delivery. They observed two types of uterine contractility. The first was a low-intensity, high-frequency pattern referred to as "Alvarez waves." This rhythmic low-intensity contraction pattern was believed to represent asynchronized local uterine activity. Alvarez and Caldeyro-Barcia [1] found this contraction pattern to be almost continuously recorded but usually not perceived. The second pattern was that of lower-frequency, higher-intensity (10–15 mm Hg) contractions. These contractions were generally painless but often palpable and are commonly referred to as "Braxton-Hicks" contractions. These higher-intensity contractions were noted to increase in frequency as labor approaches, gradually replacing the low-intensity and high-frequency contractility. Over an approximate 2-week period of time before the onset of active labor, contraction frequency and intensity both increased, which Alvarez and Caldeyro-Barcia [1] referred to as "prelabor synchronization of uterine activity." Caldeyro-Barcia reported that uterine contractions of less than 20 mm Hg are generally not perceived or palpable by the patient herself. Between 20 and 30 mm Hg patients are usually able to perceive their contractions by abdominal palpation but generally do not identify the contraction as painful until it exceeds approximately 30 mm Hg.

In 1954 Reynolds and colleagues [2] used a multichannel external toco-dynamometer to describe normal uterine contractility in the third trimester. Monitoring patients at 2-week intervals from 27 to 28 weeks' gestation Reynolds and colleagues [2] demonstrated a progressive increase in the frequency of major contractions as pregnancy advanced, most evident after the 34th week. They also demonstrated the development of "fundal dominance" [2]. Early in gestation, pressures measured over the middle and lower uterine segments exceeded those in the fundus. Later in gestation, however, pressures measured over the fundus had the greatest intensity creating a pressure gradient directed toward the lower uterine segment. In 1994, Moore and colleagues [3] performed ambulatory uterine contraction monitoring in 109 low-risk women who ultimately delivered at term. These women underwent 24-hour recording sessions twice weekly between 20 and 40 weeks' gestation. Uterine contraction frequency increased progressively with gestational age yielding mean frequencies very similar to those recorded by Reynolds and colleagues [2] 40 years previously. Statistical evaluation of the uterine contractility data revealed that the 95th percentile confidence limit was 1.3 contractions per hour at 21 to 24 weeks, 2.9 contractions per hour at 28 to 32 weeks, and 4.9 contractions per hour at 38 to 40 weeks. Among these low-risk women, 73% of the almost 72,000 hours of uterine contraction monitoring revealed no contractions and three or fewer contractions per hour were recorded 96% of the time. Also of interest, 67% of the recorded contractions after 24 weeks' gestation occurred at night, whereas maternal rest and sexual activity had small but measurable effects on contraction frequency [3]. Nageotte and colleagues [4] reviewed the uterine activity that was recorded during antenatal fetal assessment tests performed on 2446 patients using a single-channel external tocodynamometer. These investigators found that maximum uterine activity increased 4.7% per week between 30 and 44 weeks' gestation. They noted that women who delivered earlier than 38 weeks' gestation had more contractions at earlier gestational ages than did those who delivered at either 38 to 41 weeks or after 41 weeks' gestation. Most significantly, they noted a crescendo of uterine activity occurring 48 to 72 hours before the onset of labor, be it preterm, term, or postterm. Zahn [5] also demonstrated a progressive rise in uterine contraction frequency over the last trimester of pregnancy among normal ambulatory pregnant women. Before the 30th week of gestation the maximum uterine contraction frequency was approximately 2 per hour, whereas after the 30th week the mean contraction frequency was approximately 4 per hour. Zahn [5] defined normal and abnormal uterine contraction frequencies as being less than or greater than the 97th percentile confidence limits. Pathologic contraction frequencies (>97% cervical length) were more than three per hour between 26 and 28 weeks, more than four per hour between 28 and 30 weeks, and more than five per hour between 30 and 33 weeks [5]. Araki [6] found almost identical results in another series of normal pregnant women monitored on an ambulatory basis. They defined normal uterine contractility as being less than 90th percentile confidence limit. In Araki's [6] study, the critical thresholds for normal versus pathologic uterine contractility were greater than three per hour at 26 to 28 weeks, greater than four per hour at 30 weeks, greater than five per hour at 32 weeks, and greater than seven per hour at 34 to 36 weeks [6].

A final characteristic of normal uterine activity is that of diurnal variation. In the previously cited study by Moore and colleagues [3], two thirds of the contractions were recorded in the evening, whereas Zahn [5] identified an increase in uterine contractility between 10 PM and 2 AM among 54 normal women performing continuous 24-hour tocodynamometry. Zahn [5] also identified decreased uterine contractility in the early morning hours. Germain and colleagues [7] followed 19 women from 26 weeks until delivery hospitalizing them for a 24-hour period of external tocodynamometry every 2 weeks. Those patients delivering at term demonstrated a nocturnal surge in uterine contractility between 4 and 7 AM, whereas those delivering preterm showed an initial nocturnal surge of uterine activity that disappeared a little over 3 weeks before delivery. In 1982, Schwenzer and colleagues [8] described a circadian pattern of uterine contractions in resting pregnant women. They identified two peaks of uterine contractility. The first and most prominent occurred between 11 PM and 3 AM, whereas the second was between 11 AM and 1 PM. Similar to the findings of Zahn [5], Schwenzer and colleagues [8] noticed decreased uterine contractility between 3 AM and 9 AM. Schwenzer and colleagues [8] also noted that women laboring preterm seemed to lose this diurnal pattern characteristic of normal pregnancy.

It seems that normal pregnancy is characterized by almost continuous low-intensity uterine contractility with intermittent but infrequent contractions that typically range between 10 and 20 mm Hg in intensity. During an approximate 2-week prelabor period the uterus demonstrates an increased frequency of mild- to moderate-intensity contractions that is also associated with the development of fundal dominance. There is a normal circadian pattern of uterine contractility highest in the late evening and early morning hours and lower in the later morning. Patients who have preterm labor have a disruption of this normal diurnal pattern.

Abnormal uterine contractility

Bruns and colleagues [9] in 1957 described excess uterine contractility early in pregnancy among women who ultimately delivered prematurely. Using intermittent single-channel external tocodynamometry they noted that excessive uterine contractility preceded the onset of preterm labor and birth by several weeks. In describing their "perinatal concept" in 1973, Aubry and Pennington [10] reported similar findings in women who later developed preterm labor noting increased uterine contractility weeks before its clinical onset. In 1983, Bell [11] performed external tocodynamometry on 14 patients for 1 hour every 2 weeks and observed that women who later developed preterm labor between 29 and 32 weeks had an increase in the number of greater intensity contractions ($\geq$15 mm Hg) between 20 and 28 weeks of gestation. Bell [11] termed this finding "the premature synchronization" of uterine contractility.

Using a newly developed HUAM device in 1986, Katz and colleagues [12] in San Francisco monitored 34 women at high risk for preterm birth for 30 to 60 minutes four times daily. Seventeen of the women delivered before 35 weeks' gestation, whereas the other 17 labored at term. Between 22 and 35 weeks' gestation, but most pronounced after 30 weeks, there were significant differences in contraction frequency between women who delivered before 37 weeks and those who delivered at term. The mean hourly contraction frequencies per gestational week for the women who delivered preterm ranged from just over two per hour at 22 weeks to greater than five per hour by 34 weeks. Those women who delivered at term never exceeded two contractions per hour at any time between 22 and 36 weeks. When hourly uterine contraction frequencies were assessed during the 7 days before the clinical diagnosis of preterm labor there was a distinct secondary rise in uterine activity 24 to 48 hours preceding the diagnosis. In Katz' and colleagues [12] selected high-risk cohort of women with previous preterm birth, multiple gestations, uterine anomalies, and diethylstilbestrol exposure, persistent uterine contractions at a frequency of greater than four per hour between 30 and 34 weeks predicted an 80% likelihood of preterm labor.

Bentley and colleagues [13] also recorded uterine contractions in 105 women at high risk for preterm delivery and categorized them by whether or not preterm labor was ultimately diagnosed. These investigators noted that women who had four or more contractions per hour after institution of rest and hydration were much more likely to develop preterm labor than those who had fewer than four contractions per hour. Using a four contraction per hour threshold they identified 70% of the patients who developed preterm labor with a specificity of 80% and a negative predictive value of 68% [13]. In another interesting study, Main and colleagues [14] performed uterine tocodynamometry for 1 hour on 139 low-risk women between 28 and 32 weeks' gestation while in the waiting room before their prenatal visit. Excessive uterine activity identified 12 (75%) of the 16 women who subsequently developed preterm labor. The incidence of preterm labor was 3.5% in the patients with less than or equal to four contractions an hour at each of their monitoring sessions, whereas the incidence was 26.5% if greater than or equal to five contractions per hour were monitored at any session. As a result, the specificity of intermittent uterine activity monitoring in this low-risk cohort was 79%, its positive predictive value was 32%, and its negative predictive value was 96% [14].

The increased risk of prematurity among multifetal gestations has been frequently ascribed to increased uterine contractility. Using intramyometrial pressure monitoring, Alvarez and Caldeyro-Barcia [1] demonstrated an increased frequency of lower-intensity contractions associated with uterine overdistention. Using external tocodynamometry, 22 singleton pregnancies and 18 twin gestations were monitored for 2 hours a day over a 12-week period in the second half of pregnancy [15]. Uterine contraction frequencies were increased among the twin pregnancies at all gestational ages studied. In another study by the same investigators, twin gestations between 24 and 36 weeks' gestation that experienced preterm labor had significantly higher mean hourly contraction frequencies compared with women with twins who labored at term [16]. Interestingly, triplet gestations did not show a similar increase in contraction frequency when comparing those who labored preterm with those who delivered at term, although the sample size was small [16].

There has been only limited study of the low-amplitude high-frequency uterine contraction pattern previously referred to as "Alvarez waves." These so-called "Alvarez waves" are defined as uterine activity with an intensity of less than 5 mm Hg occurring at a frequency of every 1 to 2 minutes. Alvarez and Caldeyro-Barcia [1] believed this pattern of uterine activity represented local contractions occurring randomly in different parts of the uterus, which they described as "uterine fibrillation" [1]. Although this pattern of uterine activity is generally not perceived by women it can be detected by external tocodynamome-try. The significance of the low-amplitude high-frequency contraction pattern is uncertain. Warkentin [17] described low-amplitude high-frequency contractions as accounting for 70% to 80% of the total contractions recorded during the course of a normal pregnancy. Based solely on its ubiquitous nature Warkentin [17] concluded that low-amplitude high-frequency contractility was not associated with preterm labor or poor outcome. Creasy [18] concluded that the low-amplitude high-frequency contraction pattern is a prodromal event leading to the development of more synchronous contractions of greater intensity and sub-sequently to preterm labor.

Newman and colleagues [19] studied the low-amplitude high-frequency con-traction pattern to determine its clinical relevance. Among 142 high-risk women undergoing daily uterine activity monitoring, the women who ultimately developed preterm labor demonstrated the low-amplitude high-frequency pattern more often than did the women who delivered at term (13.5% versus 9.2%; $P < .01$). Parity and gestational age did not seem to affect the occurrence of this pattern but it was more prevalent in multifetal gestations. Tocolytic therapy reduced the amount of time spent in this low-amplitude high-frequency pattern by 50% but did not eliminate it. Kawarabayashi and colleagues [20] studied 6363 cardiotocographs obtained from 578 patients. They observed the presence of low-amplitude high-frequency contractility in 7.5% of the patients studied. They noticed a decrease in the rate of low-amplitude high-frequency contractility as pregnancy progressed as originally described by Alvarez and Caldeyro-Barcia [1], but noted an increase in low-amplitude high-frequency activity in 42.3% of patients with premature labor. These investigators concluded that increased low-amplitude high-frequency activity was associated with preterm birth and poor obstetric outcomes. Low-amplitude high-frequency activity may indicate the presence of a state of high excitability and poor coordination of the uterine muscles that precedes development of the necessary coordination to generate larger more intense phasic contractions [20].

In a recently published article in the *New England Journal of Medicine* Iams and colleagues [21] investigated the validity of uterine contraction frequency as a predictor of spontaneous preterm birth in a cohort of risk-enhanced singleton gestations participating in a large National Institutes of Health–sponsored preterm prediction study. The 297 singleton gestations were recruited before 24 weeks' gestation with a history of prior preterm birth, second-trimester bleeding, or with no risk factors (N = 52). In the aforementioned study, women performed uterine activity monitoring at least 2 days per week for 2 hours, once during the morning and once during the afternoon. Monitoring was continued until delivery or until 37 weeks' gestation and the uterine monitoring data were blinded to the care providers. As a result of risk enhancement 97 of the singletons (32.6%) delivered between 29 and 36 weeks' gestations. Although a large percentage of the monitoring strips recorded no contractions (79%) the investigation did identify a significant increase in uterine contraction frequency associated with advancing gestational age (between 4 PM and 4 AM) and in women who spontaneously delivered before 35 weeks' gestation. Unfortunately, receiver-operator character-istic curve analysis of the data could not identify a threshold value of uterine contraction frequency that efficiently predicted the risk of spontaneous preterm delivery [21]. Between 27 and 28 weeks' gestation greater than or equal to four contractions per hour in the evening had sensitivity and a positive predictive value of only 28% and 23%, respectively, for spontaneous preterm birth less than or equal to 35 week's gestation. It is noted, however, that uterine contraction frequency was similar in both its sensitivity and positive predictive value to fetal fibronectin, endovaginal cervical length measurements, and digital cervical ex-amination among the singleton gestations.

It is clear that premature birth is multifactorial with numerous predisposing factors and pathophysiologic mechanisms. Increased uterine contractility, how-ever, seems to be a final common pathway to prematurity. As a result, most women who are destined to labor prematurely demonstrate an increase uterine contraction frequency for weeks to months before the clinical diagnosis. Unfor-tunately, this baseline increase in uterine contraction frequency is not substan-tial enough to make it a reliable or efficient predictor of preterm delivery risk. There is, however, a secondary and significant increase in uterine contractility, which occurs in the 24 to 8 hours preceding the clinical diagnosis of preterm labor. This secondary crescendo of uterine activity suggests the possible clinical use of HUAM to make an earlier diagnosis of preterm labor at a time when tocolysis can be more effective in prolonging the pregnancy and in reducing neonatal morbidity and mortality.

Potential interventions

Clinical trials investigating the use of uterine contraction monitoring for the early diagnosis of preterm labor have generally involved four different study methodologies: (1) self-identification of preterm labor signs or symptoms, (2) frequent perinatal nursing contact, (3) HUAM alone, or (4) frequent perinatal nursing contact with HUAM. Self-identification of preterm labor signs and symptoms as a primary clinical intervention was first described by Herron and colleagues [22] in the San Francisco Preterm Birth Prevention Program in the early 1980s. This intervention consisted of educating patients regarding maternal symptoms suggestive of preterm labor; instruction in self-palpation for uterine contractions; frequent (every 1–2 weeks) office visits with cervical examination; and 24-hours-a-day, 7-days-per-week access to the office or the labor and de-livery unit for emergency evaluation of potential preterm labor. Although this approach to preterm birth prevention was not as successful in subsequent studies as it was in the initial San Francisco pilot, it established a component of what has become standard care for women at increased risk of preterm birth.

The concern with self-detection of preterm labor signs and symptoms is highlighted by the initial work of Alvarez and Caldeyro-Barcia [1]. Most prelabor uterine activity remains below the threshold of effective maternal identification [1]. Contractions with intensity of less than 20 mm Hg are probably not perceptible to the patient, either by abdominal palpation or by the appreciation of discomfort or pain. Newman and colleagues [23] compared the accuracy of maternal self-perception with HUAM in 44 women at high risk for preterm birth. During the study period more than 9500 preterm contractions were recorded, but the study participants correctly identified only 15% ± 21% of these contractions. There was significant individual variation with a range of 0% to 78% but overall maternal accuracy was poor. Only five patients (11%) correctly identified greater than or equal to 50% of their contractions, whereas 54.5% identified fewer than 10% and 22.7% (10 patients) never detected any of their contractions. There was also a high frequency of false perception with almost 1000 self-reported contractions that were unconfirmed by simultaneous uterine activity monitoring. It is also confirmed that women who identified more than 50% of their contractions also had the highest rates of false perception suggesting a shotgun approach to self-detection. Study subject's perception of their uterine activity did not improve with gestational age or the duration of monitoring but was significantly worse in those with twin gestations [23]. The higher frequency of lower-intensity contractions in multifetal gestations combined with a greater amount of fetal activity and general maternal discomfort was believed to be responsible for this reduced perceptive accuracy in multiples.

In a follow-up study Newman and colleagues [24] enrolled 79 women hospitalized with preterm premature rupture of the membranes between 26 and 34 weeks' gestation who were undergoing expectant management. All patients were initially educated regarding self-detection of preterm labor signs and symptoms. Each morning, patients underwent 1 hour of uterine tocodynamometry that was blinded to the patient and the care providers. They were simultaneously asked to report their subjective perception of uterine activity. The study group underwent a total of 419 days of uterine activity monitoring and most of the recordings (78%) revealed fewer than four contractions per hour. On 97.6% of these days the patients' subjective assessment of uterine activity agreed with the electronic uterine monitoring that they were indeed having fewer than four contractions per hour. On 91 days, however, greater than or equal to four contractions were recorded by the electronic monitoring. On 66 (73%) of those days the patient's simultaneous subjective perception was that she was still having fewer than four contractions per hour. Ultimately, each of the 79 patients entered spontaneous preterm labor and in 58 (73%) of those cases uterine activity was objectively increased ($\geq$ four contractions per hour) within 24 hours of the onset of labor. Maternal self-detection of uterine activity was significantly less likely (32%; $P < .01$) to identify this crescendo in uterine activity compared with the uterine activity monitoring [24].

The largest study of this type involved over 70,000 uterine activity records in 778 patients receiving HUAM [25]. Monitored women were asked to mark using an electronic signaling device whenever they palpated or perceived a uterine contraction. Once again, the accuracy of maternal perception of prelabor uterine activity was poor with the mean percentage of correct identification being only 14.1% per patient. The patients also signaled the presence of contractions that were not electronically recorded 40.3% of the time. This is consistent with the clinical experience of patients coming for unscheduled visits because of the false perception of preterm labor contractions.

This high failure rate in the detection of prelabor uterine activity by women relying on self-palpation as their primary mechanism of surveillance raises obvious concern. Self-palpation of uterine activity is probably aided by both maternal assessments of preterm labor symptoms and by frequent office visits. Among 42 women with confirmed preterm labor in a randomized clinical trial by Martin and colleagues [26], uterine contractions were the initiator of contact in 31% of patients. Patient-reported signs and symptoms led to the diagnosis of preterm labor in 24% of the patients, whereas 26% of the patients had both. Importantly, 19% of the patients were diagnosed by physician evaluation during a routine office visit or during an unscheduled visit for issues other than those related to preterm labor. Other studies have also shown the importance of patient-identified signs and symptoms of preterm labor [27,28]. Unfortunately, a prospective evaluation of preterm labor signs and symptoms by Iams [29] has confirmed what is intuitively appreciated: that these signs and symptoms lack significant positive predictive value or specificity.

Another methodologic approach to preterm birth prevention is that of frequent perinatal nursing contact. This approach builds on the patient education intervention described previously by providing frequent, and in many cases daily, contact between the at-risk patient and a specialized perinatal nurse. The perinatal nurses support the educational component by systematically questioning the patients regarding signs and symptoms of preterm labor and their subjective uterine contraction frequency based on self-palpation. In addition, the perinatal nurse reinforces the educational objectives and assesses patient compliance with physician-directed therapies or restrictions. A less obvious benefit of the perinatal nurse is the rapport that she develops with the patient and how that rapport can lend itself to stress reduction, emotional support, and encouragement. The perinatal nurse also serves as a liaison between the patient and the primary care provider and is dedicated only to serving a cadre of patients and is without other clinical duties. The perinatal nurse frequently becomes a patient confidant and is in an excellent position to be an intermediary with the physician regarding patient requests or concerns and noncompliance issues. Another important aspect of the perinatal nursing contact is its availability on a 24-hours-per-day, 7-days-per-week basis so that the patient can be in immediate contact with her care providers by telephone rather than having to go to the office, emergency room, or labor and delivery unit. An elegant description of the potential benefits engendered by having the perinatal nurse in frequent contact with the high-risk patient was provided by Merkatz and Merkatz in 1991 [30].

The HUAM is approved by the Food and Drug Administration (FDA) as a device capable of detecting preterm labor. The device consists of a Smyth Guard-Ring tocodynamometer as opposed to the typical plunger-type device used for monitoring labor contractions at term [31]. The Smyth Guard-Ring tocodyna-mometer has been compared side-by-side with traditional external contraction monitors and simultaneous intrauterine pressure catheters. The Guard-Ring device performed well in detecting contractions confirmed by the intrauterine pressure catheter and was substantially better than the traditional monitoring devices at detecting contractions before 32 weeks' gestation [32,33]. This is of critical importance because neither contraction duration, nor amplitude, nor rhythmicity differentiates those patients with true preterm labor from those with spurious labor. Contraction frequency was the only component of prelabor uterine activity that correlated well with ultimately confirmed preterm labor [34]. In most protocols the HUAM device is used to monitor uterine contractility at home for 1 hour in the evening and for 1 hour the following morning. The patient is then called and the uterine contractility data are retrieved by telephone modem and the number of contractions counted. Contractions are usually identified by a typical appearance and duration of greater than 40 seconds. Patients with greater than or equal to four contractions per hour are usually asked to hydrate, void, assume bed rest in the lateral recumbent position, remonitor for 1 hour, and send in a second HUAM strip. If excessive uterine activity is still present the health care provider is contacted and further plans for evaluation of the patient are made.

With the exception of selected clinical trials, HUAM is usually not performed in isolation but rather as a comprehensive system involving both the uterine activity monitoring along with perinatal nursing support. In addition to retrieving the uterine contractility data, the perinatal nurse assesses the patient for signs or symptoms associated with preterm labor and the patient's perception of those contractions as painful or not. The contributions of the perinatal nurse described previously are coincidental with the telephone contact to retrieve the uterine monitoring data. In a comprehensive system of preterm birth prevention, the patient-reported symptoms and the electronically recorded uterine activity are synergistic in making an early diagnosis of preterm labor. Iams and colleagues [27] reported that nearly 50% of the cases of confirmed preterm labor occurred in patients who had both excess uterine contractility by HUAM and reported symptoms of preterm labor. The diagnosis of preterm labor would be delayed in approximately 25% of cases if uterine activity data and patient-reported symptomatology were not considered simultaneously [27].

The simultaneous assessment of an individual patient's signs and symptoms during the daily perinatal nursing telephone call along with objective uterine activity monitoring complemented by 24-hours-per-day, 7-days-per-week availability are believed to be critical factors in the early diagnosis of preterm labor. In the following sections, examples of randomized trials are presented comparing HUAM augmented by daily perinatal nursing contact versus standard preterm birth prevention education with less frequent perinatal nursing contact (Table 1); comprehensive perinatal nursing contact with and without HUAM (Table 2); HUAM with frequent perinatal nursing contact versus frequent perinatal nursing contact with sham HUAM versus standard preterm birth prevention education alone (Table 3); HUAM alone without perinatal nursing support versus standard

Table 1

Prospective randomized trial comparing HUAM and daily PNC with standard preterm birth prevention education augmented by twice weekly PNC

	HUAM plus daily PNC	Standard education plus twice weekly PNC
Number	34	33
Preterm labor (%)	24 (71)	22 (67)
Gestational age at PTL (wk)	27.9 ± 2.4	29.4 ± 2.7
Cervical dilatation ≤2 cm (%)	18 (75)	7 (32)[a]
Pregnancy prolongation (wk)	8.2 ± 2.7	4.2 ± 2.9[b]
PTB <37 wk (%)	5 (15)	15 (45)[b]
Birth weight <2500 g (%)	2 of 45 (4)	12 of 41 (29)[b]
NICU admission (%)	7 of 45 (16)	18 of 41 (44)[b]

Patients were at high risk for PTB because of a prior PTB (42), multiple gestation (18), or other indication (7).

Abbreviations: HUAM, home uterine activity monitoring; PNC, perinatal nursing contact; PTB, preterm birth; PTL, preterm labor.

   [a] $P < .01$.

   [b] $P < .05$.

Data from Morrison JC, Martin Jr JN, Martin RW, et al. Prevention of preterm birth by ambulatory assessment of uterine activity: a randomized study. Am J Obstet Gynecol 1987;156:536–43; with permission.

preterm birth prevention education (Table 4); and daily perinatal nursing contact versus weekly perinatal nursing contact versus daily perinatal nursing contact plus HUAM (Table 5). Most of these illustrative examples of various study designs have been emulated by other investigators with remarkably consistent results. The likelihood of progressive cervical dilatation or spontaneous rupture of the membranes resulting in early delivery increases dramatically with cervical dilatation greater than or equal to 3 cm at the internal os. In contrast, earlier

Table 2

Prospective randomized trial comparing comprehensive PNC with and without HUAM

	HUAM plus daily PNC	Standard education plus 5/wk PNC
Number	184	82
Preterm labor (%)	66 (36)	28 (34)
Gestational age at PTL (wk)	32.1 ± 3.3	31.5 ± 3.8
Pregnancy prolongation (wk)	7.4 ± 1.2	8 ± 4.4
PTB <37 wk (%)	67 (36)	35 (43)
Gestational age at delivery (wk)	35.5 ± 2.9	35.6 ± 2.5
Birth weight (g)	2769 ± 780	2726 ± 665

Patients were at high risk for PTB caused by a prior PTB (173), multiple gestations (41), or other indications (94). No differences were statistically significant.

Abbreviations: HUAM, home uterine activity monitoring; PNC, perinatal nursing contact; PTB, preterm birth; PTL, preterm labor.

Data from references [39] and [40].

Table 3
Prospective randomized trial comparing HUAM with frequent PNC versus frequent PNC with sham HUAM versus standard preterm birth prevention education without PNC

	HUAM plus 5/wk PNC	Sham HUAM plus 5/wk PNC	Standard education
Number	120	127	143
Preterm labor (%)	49 (41)	47 (38)	53 (37)
Gestational age at PTL (wk)	30.1 ± 0.6	29.6 ± 0.6	29.6 ± 0.9
Cervical dilatation ≤2 cm (%)	96 (80)	97 (76)	41 (28)[a]
Pregnancy prolongation (d)	36.9 ± 4.9	36.1 ± 5.4	7 ± 4.2[b]
PTB <36 wk (%)	28 (23)	32 (25)	64 (45)[b]
Gestational age at delivery (wk)	35.4 ± 0.7	34.7 ± 0.8	30.9 ± 0.6[b]
Birth weight (g)	2813 ± 821	2709 ± 910	2550 ± 962[a]
Birth weight <2500 g (%)	34 (29)	40 (33)	60 (42)[a]
NICU stay (d)	7.2 ± 1	7.7 ± 1.6	11.3 ± 1.2

Patients were at high risk for PTB caused by a prior PTB (number not specified) and multiple gestations (189).

Abbreviations: HUAM, home uterine activity monitoring; PNC, perinatal nursing contact; PTB, preterm birth; PTL, preterm labor.

  [a] $P<.05$ HUAM/sham HUAM vs standard education.

  [b] $P<.01$ HUAM/sham HUAM vs standard education.

Data from Dyson DC, Crites YM, Ray DA, et al. Prevention of preterm birth in high risk patients: the role of education and pronder contact vs home uterine monitoring. Am J Obstet Gynecol 1991;164: 756–62; with permission.

diagnosis allows successful tocolytic treatment with the opportunity to prolong the pregnancy by several weeks (3–6) rather than a few days.

Clinical trials of home uterine activity monitoring

Clinical trials 1986 to 1989

The initial clinical trials using HUAM were performed by Katz and colleagues [35] in San Francisco. This first investigation was a nonrandomized comparison of 76 high-risk patients compared with a like number of matched controls. The study was performed in a nonrandomized fashion because of a limited number of available monitors. Inclusion criteria included a prior history of preterm birth, multiple gestations, uterine anomaly, incompetent cervix with a cerclage, or diethylstilbestrol exposure. The control group was matched for indication, gestational age, and parity. The monitored group received twice-daily HUAM combined with daily perinatal nursing assessment by telephone, whereas the matched control group received standardized preterm birth prevention education and instruction in self-palpation of uterine activity. The incidence of preterm labor was not different between the monitored (51%) and matched control group (45%); however, all of the preterm labor patients in the HUAM group were candidates for tocolytic therapy, whereas only 35% of the preterm labor patients in the matched control group were candidates. Patients were not believed to be

Table 4
Prospective randomized trial comparing HUAM without PNC versus standard preterm birth prevention education

	HUAM / no PNC	Standard education / no PNC
Number	198	179
Preterm labor (%)	43 (25)	39 (24)
Gestational age at PTL (wk)	32.9 ± 5.2	32.9 ± 2.9
Cervical dilatation ≤2 cm (%)	31 (73)	11 (28)[a]
Cervical dilatation mean (cm)	1.4 ± 1.3	2.5 ± 1.5[a]
Pregnancy prolongation (wk)	3.7 ± 3.8	2 ± 2.9[b]
Gestational age at delivery (wk)	36.6 ± 2.4	34.9 ± 3.2[a]
Birth weight (g)	2934 ± 708	2329 ± 733[a]
Birth weight <2500 g (%)	8 (19)	25 (63)[a]
NICU admissions (%)	5 (12)	13 (33)[b]
All women randomized		
PTB <37 wk (%)	22 of 164 (13)	35 of 154 (23)[b]
PTB <31 wk (%)	2 of 164 (1)	9 of 154 (6)[b]
Birth weight <2500 g (%)	19 of 155 (12)	37 of 142 (26)[a]
Birth weight <2000 g (%)	9 of 155 (6)	20 of 142 (14)[b]
Birth weight <1500 g (%)	0 of 155 (0)	7 of 42 (5)[a]
NICU admission	17 of 164 (10)	32 of 142 (23)[b]

Patients were at high risk for PTB caused by a prior PTB (186), multiple gestation (38), or other indications (101). Obstetrican and neonatal outcomes are also shown for all women randomized.
Abbreviations: HUAM, home uterine activity monitoring; PNC, perinatal nursing contact; PTB, preterm birth; PTL, preterm labor.
   [a] $P < .005$.
   [b] $P < .05$.
Data from Mou SM, Sunjerji SG, Gall S, et al. Multicenter randomized clinical trial of home uterine activity monitoring for detection of preterm labor. Am J Obstet Gynecol 1991;165:858–66; and Corwin MJ, Mou SM, Sunjerji, et al. Multicenter randomized clinical trial of home uterine activity monitoring: pregnance outcomes for all women randomized. Am J Obstet Gynecol 1996;175:1281–5; with permission.

candidates for tocolytic therapy if the cervical dilatation was greater than 4 cm or if the patient had experienced preterm premature rupture of the membranes. As a result of the earlier diagnosis of preterm labor in the HUAM group only 8 (12%) of 76 patients delivered before 37 weeks' gestation as opposed to 31 (41%) of 76 ($P < .001$) in the matched control group.

Simultaneously, Katz and colleagues [36] were also performing a second nonrandomized cohort trial of HUAM among women who had developed preterm labor during the current pregnancy and who had been successfully tocolyzed. Sixty women received twice-daily HUAM and daily perinatal nursing contact on discharge from the hospital and were compared with a matched control group also of 60 women who were discharged following instruction on the signs and symptoms of recurrent preterm labor and the technique of self-palpation of uterine activity. In both the HUAM group and the matched control group, oral terbutaline was adjusted to maintain the uterine contraction frequency at less than four per hour based either on objective electronic uterine contraction monitoring

Table 5
Prospective randomized trial comparing weekly PNC versus daily PNC versus daily PNC with HUAM

	Weekly PNC	Daily PNC	Daily PNC plus HUAM
Number	798	796	828
Preterm labor <35 wk (%)	22 (2)	23 (2)	27 (3)
Gestational age at PTL (wk)	31 ± 2.8	31 ± 2	30.7 ± 3.9
Cervical dilatation ≤2 cm (%)	17 (77)	18 (77)	22 (82)
Cervical dilatation mean (cm)	1.8	1.5	1.4
Pregnancy prolongation (d)	28 ± 2.4	26 ± 2.6	31 ± 2.5
Gestational age at delivery (wk)	35 ± 30	34.7 ± 3.2	35.1 ± 3.2
PTB <35 wk (%)	3 (14)	3 (13)	4 (13)
Birth weight <2500 g	26 (3)	26 (3)	28 (3)

Patients were at high risk for PTB caused by prior PTB (447), multiple gestation (838), or one of 12 other risk factors for PTB (474). No differences were statistically significant.
Abbreviations: HUAM, home uterine activity monitoring; PNC, perinatal nursing contact; PTB, preterm birth; PTL, preterm labor.
Data from Dyson DC, Danbe KH, Bamber JA, et al. Monitoring women at risk for preterm labor. N Engl J Med 1998;338:15–9; with permission.

or on subjective maternal self-palpation. Forty-six women (77%) in the HUAM group had a total of 83 episodes of recurrent preterm labor compared with 41 women (68%) in the matched control group who had 59 episodes of recurrent preterm labor. Only 4 (10%) of the 46 patients in the HUAM group with recurrent preterm labor failed tocolysis, whereas 13 (36%) of the 41 in the matched control group failed tocolysis. As a result, the frequency of term birth was significantly higher for the HUAM group (90%) compared with the matched control group (64%; $P<.05$). The mean time gained in utero for patients using HUAM and perinatal nursing contact was significantly longer (7.4 ± 3 weeks) than for those who used self-palpation (4 ± 1.2 weeks).

The first prospective randomized clinical trial evaluating HUAM was performed by Morrison and colleagues [37] at the University of Mississippi. Sixty-seven women at high risk for preterm labor (42 with a prior history of preterm birth, 18 with a multiple gestation, and 7 other) were randomized into two groups. The HUAM group (N = 34) received twice daily uterine monitoring and daily perinatal nursing contact by telephone. The control group received standard high-risk care augmented by instruction in self-palpation of uterine activity and by perinatal nursing contact by telephone twice per week (see Table 1). Both groups had access to a 24-hours-a-day, 7-days-a-week hotline if preterm labor signs or symptoms developed. A similar number of patients in each group developed preterm labor; however, those patients in the control group presented with greater mean cervical dilatation ($P<.001$) and effacement greater than 50% ($P<.01$) compared with the HUAM group. As a result, 92% of the patients in the HUAM group were considered candidates for tocolytic therapy with a mean time gained in utero of 8.2 ± 2.7 weeks compared with only 45% of the patients in the control group being candidates for tocolytic therapy with a mean time gained in utero of only 4.2 ± 2 weeks ($P<.05$). Ultimately 29 of

34 patients in the HUAM group delivered greater than or equal to 37 weeks' gestation compared with only 18 of 33 ($P < .05$) in the control group.

In 1987, Porto and colleagues [38] presented an abstract at the Society of Perinatal Obstetricians annual meeting that was unfortunately never published. The abstract reported on 129 high-risk pregnancies that were randomized between three groups. The 41 patients in group 1 received daily HUAM with perinatal nursing contact where the uterine contraction monitoring data were used for clinical management. Group 2 included 42 patients who also performed daily HUAM and received perinatal nursing contact; however, the uterine contraction monitoring data were blinded from the investigators and not used clinically. Group 3 included 46 women receiving routine high-risk care. Thirteen patients experienced preterm labor in all three groups but the likelihood of preterm delivery varied considerably. Four (31%) of 13 patients in group 1 delivered preterm compared with 6 (46%) of 13 in group 2. Both of these groups did significantly better than those in the routine care group 3 where 11 (85%) of 13 patients delivered prematurely ($P < .005$). The performance of group 2 in the Porto investigation was the first suggestion of the potential value of frequent perinatal nursing contact alone in patients at high risk for preterm birth.

Following up on the study by Porto and colleagues [38], Iams and colleagues [39,40] published two papers in 1987 and 1988 describing the first and second years of a study involving 184 women at high risk for preterm delivery (124 prior preterm birth, 13 multiple gestations, and 62 other) who were randomized to a comprehensive program of daily HUAM and perinatal nursing contact. These women were compared with 82 women at high risk for preterm delivery (49 prior preterm birth, 28 multiple gestations, and 32 other) who were educated regarding the signs and symptoms of preterm labor and the technique of self-palpation of uterine activity. In addition, the comparison group received perinatal nursing contact 5 days-per-week and had the availability of a 24-hours-a-day; 7-days-a-week hotline should signs or symptoms of preterm labor develop (see Table 2). Ultimately, 67 (36.4%) of the 184 patients in the HUAM group delivered before 37 weeks' gestation compared with 35 (42.7%) of 82 in the control group, which was not a statistically significant difference. Similarly, there were no differences in the rate of birth less than 35 weeks' gestation, birth weight, or prolongation of pregnancy. Significantly, however, the authors noted an overall decrease in the rate of preterm birth for all patients between the first (46%) and second (30%) year of the trial ($P < .01$). The authors believed that the frequent contact between the perinatal nurse and the patient resulted in this improvement. Increased attention to the patient-reported signs and symptoms of preterm labor combined with heightened physician awareness ultimately decreased the number of preterm labor patients presenting with advanced cervical change and consequently they were able to decrease the preterm birth rate for the entire cohort.

In response to these studies the American College of Obstetricians and Gynecologists (ACOG) published a committee opinion on HUAM in 1989 [41]. The committee opinion was that HUAM had not been shown to add independently to the value of frequent provider-initiated telephone contact. ACOG recommended that use of HUAM remain investigational while awaiting further prospective control trials. In the meantime, HUAM could not yet be recommended for routine clinical use. The Diagnostic Therapeutic Technology Assessment committee also evaluated HUAM in 1989 and concluded that a system of HUAM, including daily nursing contact, could lower the preterm birth rate in high-risk women [42]. They recommended further study to determine the relative contributions of the monitored uterine activity data versus daily nursing contact. Most of the panel (61%) believed that the safety of HUAM had been established, but only 14% of the consultants believed that the effectiveness of HUAM had been established.

Clinical trials 1990 to 1993

Up until this point in time all the studies of HUAM had been performed at a single institution. The first multicentered prospective randomized trial was performed by Hill and colleagues [43] in 299 women at high risk for preterm delivery with similar indications as the studies previously described. Women were randomized to receive HUAM with daily perinatal nursing contact (N = 155) or high-risk care enhanced by preterm birth prevention education and more frequent prenatal visits but no daily nursing contact or electronic uterine contraction monitoring (N = 144). Once again there was no significant difference in the incidence of preterm labor; however, at the time that preterm labor was diagnosed the HUAM group had fewer patients with a cervix greater than 4 cm dilated (12% versus 0%) and greater than 2 cm but less than or equal to 4 cm (34% versus 19%) compared with the control group ($P < .005$). Not surprisingly, with these differences in cervical dilatation the preterm delivery rate in the HUAM group was only 42% compared with 65% in the preterm birth prevention education-enhanced care group ($P < .02$).

In 1991, Dyson and colleagues [28] reported on the results of three separate preterm birth prevention interventions from the Kaiser Health Care System in California [28]. Dyson and colleagues enrolled women with either high-risk singleton pregnancies (N = 201) or twins (N = 189) into one of three treatment groups. Group 1 was a program of standard high-risk care with weekly prenatal visits after 24 weeks' gestation. Patients enrolled in this group received weekly educational sessions regarding the signs and symptoms of preterm labor and were taught self-palpation of uterine activity. Group 2 received the same program of preterm birth prevention education and instruction in self-palpation of uterine activity and was provided with a HUAM. These patients were contacted by a dedicated perinatal nurse five times per week and were questioned about preterm labor symptoms and their frequency of uterine contractions by self-palpation. These patients performed HUAM but the uterine activity data generated by the monitor was not available to the care providers (sham). Group 3 received the same educational program as group 2 and was also contacted five times per week by a dedicated perinatal nurse; however, the HUAM data generated by these patients were used for clinical management (see Table 3). A threshold of greater than or equal to six contractions per hour was used as a trigger point for further monitoring or physician assessment. The rates of preterm labor were not different in any of the three groups. The patients in group 3 (preterm birth prevention education, frequent perinatal nursing contact, and HUAM) had less cervical dilatation at the time of preterm labor diagnosis, a lower rate of delivery less than 36 weeks' gestation, a greater gestational age at delivery, and more days gained in utero compared with the standard preterm birth prevention education group 1. The patients in group 2 who received the same program of preterm birth prevention education as group 1 but were augmented by frequent perinatal nursing contact with sham HUAM also had significant improvements in all the same outcomes compared with the standard care controls. The only benefits specific to the clinical use of HUAM were among the twin gestations. The rate of NICU admission among the twin gestations fell from 43.9% in women relying on education and self-palpation along with perinatal nursing contact but sham HUAM (group 2) to 27.9% for group 3 with active HUAM ($P<.05$). There was also a reduction in the neonatal hospital stay from 10.2 to 5.6 days comparing the sham versus active monitored twins. Among the twin gestation cohort, both group 2 and group 3 did substantially better than the standard high-risk care group 1 without the benefit of frequent perinatal nursing contact or HUAM. The differences among the singleton gestation cohort were not as remarkable, which the author attributed to the sample size and the lower risk of preterm birth. Although there were no significant differences between the singleton groups receiving frequent perinatal nursing contact, both of these groups again did better than group 1 receiving standard high-risk care without perinatal nursing contact or HUAM.

Another prospective randomized trial underscoring the importance of control group selection was performed by Blondel and colleagues [44] in France in 1992. They compared a group of 84 women at risk for preterm birth using HUAM and daily telephone contact by a nurse midwife compared with 84 other high-risk women who received home visits by nurse midwives. In this study there were no differences in the frequency of preterm delivery between the two groups (32% versus 22%; odds ratio 1.7; 95% confidence interval [CI], 0.9–3.5). It is difficult to interpret this lack of difference between the two treatment groups because the control group intervention of home visits by nurse midwives is not available to a large percentage of similar high-risk obstetric patients in the United States.

Late in 1991 the National Institutes of Health convened a HUAM workshop whose proceedings were published [45]. The workshop concluded that a comprehensive program of twice-daily HUAM in high-risk women in conjunction with daily perinatal nursing contact resulted in a marked increase in the number of monitored patients who were candidates for tocolysis and a marked decrease in the rate of preterm birth. They also found no evidence that HUAM resulted in an increased frequency of diagnosed preterm labor. They noted several limitations of the available clinical trials. Namely, most of the randomized trials were of modest size, they failed to show results for women who withdrew, there were unblinded treatment assignments, and there was a confounding influence of the extra period of rest associated with HUAM. Most importantly, they emphasized the unclear relative importance of HUAM versus perinatal nursing contact. They stated, however, "in spite of these limitations, the findings that the combined nursing and monitoring program has led to a substantial reduction in preterm births in these very high risk women remains a striking, perhaps unprecedented result."

To gain approval from the FDA for the HUAM device (Genesis System; Physiologic Diagnostic Services, Atlanta, Georgia) Mou and colleagues [46] designed a multicentered prospective randomized trial involving 377 women at risk for preterm birth at three university centers. The methodology for this study was unique compared with previous investigations. The control group included 179 patients who were provided preterm birth prevention education and were instructed in self-palpation of uterine activity but received no perinatal nursing support or HUAM. The HUAM group consisted of 198 women who performed electronic uterine contraction assessment for 2 hours each day and transmitted that data to the study center, but without any perinatal nursing contact (see Table 4). The percentage of patients developing preterm labor in each group was virtually identical (24% versus 25%) as was the gestational age at which preterm labor occurred. By the time that preterm labor was diagnosed, however, the mean cervical dilatation was 1.4 cm in the HUAM group compared with 2.5 cm in patients receiving preterm birth prevention education and self-palpation instruction ($P < .0006$). At the time that preterm labor was diagnosed cervical dilatation was less than or equal to 2 cm in 73.1% of the patients performing HUAM versus only 27.8% of the patients in the education and self-palpation group ($P < .009$). Once again, as a consequence of the earlier diagnosis of preterm labor, more effective tocolysis was achieved in the HUAM group allowing a prolongation of pregnancy by 3.7 ± 3.8 weeks compared with only 2 ± 2.9 weeks in the educational and self-palpation group ($P < .02$). Other significant differences between those patients who experienced preterm labor in the HUAM group compared with the education and self-palpation group were a greater gestational age at delivery (36.6 ± 2.4 versus 34.9 ± 3.2 weeks; $P < .009$); a greater birth weight (2934 ± 708 versus 2329 ± 733 g; $P < .002$); fewer deliveries less than 2500 g (19% versus 63%; $P < .0007$); and fewer NICU admissions (5 versus 13 infants; $P < .02$). None of the infants in the HUAM group required oxygen therapy or mechanical ventilation and their average NICU stay was 10 days compared with 24.9 days for the infants of mothers in the education and self-palpation group. These results were criticized because the improved outcomes applied only to those infants whose mother's experienced preterm labor as opposed to representing differences between the entire cohorts.

The patient outcomes from the multicentered trial by Mou and colleagues [46] were re-evaluated by Corwin and colleagues [47] in 1996 in which they reported the obstetric and neonatal outcomes for all women randomized using relative risks and 95% confidence intervals. The frequency of delivery less than 37 weeks remained significant comparing the entire HUAM cohort (22 of 164) with the education and self-palpation group (35 of 154; relative risk [RR], 0.59; 95% CI, 0.37–0.95). The incidence of delivery less than 31 weeks was also significantly different between the two groups: 2 of 164 versus 9 of 154 (RR, 0.21; 95% CI, 0.05–0.95). There were also significant differences in the frequency of delivery less than 2500 g (19 of 155 versus 37 of 142; RR, 0.47; 95% CI, 0.28–0.78); delivery less than 2000 g (9 of 155 versus 20 of 142; RR, 0.41; 95% CI, 0.19–0.88); and delivery at less than 1500 g (0 of 155 versus 7 of 142). The likelihood of NICU admission was significantly different between the groups occurring in 17 infants from the HUAM group and 32 of the education and self-palpation group (RR, 0.50; 95% CI, 0.29–0.85). As a result of the Mou trial, the FDA approved the Genesis System for the early diagnosis of preterm labor in women with a previous preterm delivery after 24 weeks' gestation. The FDA did not approve the Genesis System for the prevention of preterm birth and does not advocate any single approach to the clinical care of women at risk of delivering prematurely [48].

Knuppel and colleagues [49] published a prospective randomized trial in 1990 involving twin gestations only. In this study, mothers with twins were randomly assigned to HUAM and perinatal nursing contact (N = 19) or preterm birth prevention education and instruction in the self-palpation of uterine activity without daily nursing contact or HUAM (N = 26). Women in both groups were asked to use greater than or equal to four contractions per hour as the threshold for which they should contact their primary physician. Although the incidences of preterm labor were very high there was no significant difference between the two groups (74% versus 62%). All of the women who developed preterm labor in the preterm birth prevention education and self-palpation group were greater than or equal to 3 cm at the time of diagnosis compared with only 10 of 16 patients in the HUAM group ($P < .001$). The mean cervical dilatation at the time of diagnosis was 1.6 cm in the HUAM group and 2.9 cm in the education and self-palpation group ($P < .01$). Ultimately, more patients in the education and self-palpation group (81%) delivered preterm compared with patients in the HUAM group (50%). This difference was primarily the result of failed tocolysis because of advanced cervical dilatation at the time of presentation.

In 1993, Nagey and colleagues [50] investigated HUAM in women discharged from the hospital after successful tocolysis of acute preterm labor. As in the study by Mou and colleagues [46], HUAM only was provided to 28 women, whereas 29 received routine care. Neither group had benefit of daily perinatal nursing contact nor was there access to an emergency telephone hotline. Unfortunately, 26 of the 28 patients in the HUAM group were noncompliant with the monitoring protocol at one point or another, which is substantially higher than the noncompliance rates reported in virtually all other studies. In addition, 4 of the 28 patients in the HUAM group were never discharged from the hospital and never received HUAM but remained in the analysis. When recurrent preterm labor occurred there was a trend toward less cervical dilatation and effacement in the HUAM group, but these differences were not statistically significant, nor were there any differences in the preterm delivery rates. The authors acknowledged that they needed a larger sample size to show a significant detectable difference in outcomes for the HUAM group.

Primarily as a result of these published prospective randomized trials ACOG offered a revised committee opinion regarding HUAM in 1992 [51]. ACOG concluded, as had the FDA, that HUAM is effective for the early diagnosis of preterm labor. They also concluded that the value of HUAM to identify patients at risk and to reduce the preterm birth rate is uncertain. In an additional powerful statement, however, they endorsed daily provider-initiated contact as being effective in reducing the risk of preterm birth. The following year in 1993, the US Preventive Services Task Force published an HUAM policy statement concluding that the overall evidence showed rather consistently that the combination of HUAM and frequent provider contact produces better outcomes than standard care [52]. They went on to state, however, that there is insufficient evidence to recommend for or against HUAM as a screening test for preterm labor in high-risk pregnancies, but that recommendations against its use could be made on other grounds including cost and inconvenience ("C" recommendation). A critical review of HUAM published by McLean and colleagues [53] in *Obstetrics and Gynecology Survey* also in 1993 concluded that those programs incorporating patient education, nursing care, and uterine activity monitoring for women identified as being at increased risk for preterm labor unequivocally led to improvements in the early diagnosis of preterm labor.

Clinical trials 1994 to 1997

In the latter half of the 1990s larger and more ambitious prospective randomized trials were undertaken and completed to define better the role of HUAM in women at risk for preterm birth. Despite their large size, complexity, and expense, an awareness of their flawed study design and the control group selection makes the apparently disparate findings predictable. The first of these prospective randomized trials was by Wapner and colleagues [54] who enrolled 187 patients with a history of previous preterm birth at four university sites over a 2-year period. Eighty-six women were randomized to a protocol of daily home uterine activity monitoring alone, whereas the control group of 101 women were provided with preterm birth prevention education and instructed in self-palpation of uterine activity. The incidence of preterm labor was not different between the two groups (24.4% versus 21.8%) but the cervical dilatation at the time that preterm labor was diagnosed was significantly less in the HUAM group (1.7 cm) compared with the preterm birth prevention education and self-palpation group (2.8 cm; $P < .004$). Additionally, 52.4% of the HUAM group experienced preterm labor with a cervical dilatation of less than 2 cm at diagnosis compared with only 18.2% of the education and self-palpation group ($P = .019$). Preterm labor tocolysis was successful in delaying delivery for more than 48 hours in 86% of the HUAM group with a mean prolongation of pregnancy by 21 days. Similar success was not achieved in the education and self-palpation group where 50% of the patients delivered within 48 hours of diagnosis and the mean prolongation of pregnancy was only 3 days ($P < .016$). The obstetric and neonatal outcomes favored the HUAM group among all randomized women. The mean gestational age at delivery for the HUAM group was 36.4 $\pm$ 2.5 weeks compared with the education and self-palpation group, who delivered at a mean gestational age of

35.1 ± 2.7 weeks. The mean birth weight was greater in the HUAM group (2822 ± 710 g) compared with the education and self-palpation group (2574 ± 693 g). The mean number of nursery days in the HUAM group was also reduced (4.8 ± 5.9 versus 9.8 ± 17.3 days) and more admissions to the NICU occurred among the education and self-palpation group ($P < .001$). There were only eight total NICU days in the HUAM group compared with 136 days in the unmonitored group. In terms of study design, Wapner's group emulated the methodology of Mou and colleagues [46] in that the HUAM group received only the uterine activity monitoring device. Neither group received any perinatal nursing support either by telephone or home visit. The study by Wapner and colleagues [54] demonstrated (as did Mou) that the device alone allowed earlier detection of preterm labor thereby providing an opportunity for greater pregnancy prolongation and improved obstetric and neonatal outcomes when compared with standard high-risk care.

In 1995, the Collaborative Home Uterine Monitoring Study Group [55] published another large multicentered prospective trial involving 18 sites randomizing 1292 patients over a 28-month period. Patients were enrolled based on 1 of 15 risk factors for preterm birth, although some of the indications were not strongly associated with an increased risk of prematurity. Of the enrolled patients, 842 (72.3%) completed the study. Women were randomized to one of two groups: active HUAM (N = 405) and sham HUAM (N = 437). Both groups received daily nursing contact. As with all the other prospective randomized trials the percentage of patients who developed preterm labor was not different between the two groups (24% versus 24.4%). Cervical dilatation of any degree (≤ 1, ≤ 2, or ≤ 3 cm) at the time of diagnosis of preterm labor always numerically favored the active HUAM group; however, the differences were not statistically significant. The mean cervical dilatation at the time that preterm labor was diagnosed was identical (1.6 cm) for both groups. The incidence of preterm delivery in the active HUAM group was 33% compared with 39% in the sham monitoring group (NS). Improvements in the rate of preterm delivery less than 34 weeks, birth weight less than 2500 g, NICU admission, length of neonatal hospitalization, and neonatal complications all favored the active HUAM group, but were also not significant. The study concluded that assessment of uterine contraction data was not associated with an earlier diagnosis, lower rate of preterm birth, or enhanced neonatal outcome when added to daily perinatal nursing contact. The relatively lax inclusion criteria and a higher than usual dropout rate were of concern. Another concern is that the protocol used greater than or equal to six contractions per hour as the threshold for evaluation, which is somewhat higher than most other studies have used and might allow some women to escape the earliest possible detection of their preterm labor. Most importantly, however, the study did not include a standard care group (ie, a group without daily perinatal nursing contact). The sham monitoring group does not represent what is the current standard of care for most obstetric practices in the United States.

The largest investigation of HUAM was a second study published by Dyson and colleagues [56] from the Kaiser System in Northern California, this time involving 30 centers. Over a 4-year period, 2422 pregnancies with at least 1 of

14 risk factors were randomized into one of three groups: (1) weekly contact with a perinatal nurse, (2) daily contact with a perinatal nurse, or (3) daily contact with a perinatal nurse plus HUAM (see Table 5). Women in each of the first two groups were provided with preterm birth prevention education and instructed in the self-palpation of uterine activity with an alarm threshold of six or more contractions per hour. Group 3 received the same education and daily perinatal nursing contact but also performed uterine activity monitoring during their telephone contact. The demographic characteristics, distribution of risk factors, and the incidence of preterm labor were similar between the weekly contact group (N = 798); the daily contact group (N = 796); and the HUAM group (N = 828). The mean cervical dilatation at the time of diagnosis of preterm labor was 1.8 cm in the weekly contract group, 1.5 cm in the daily contact group, and 1.4 cm in the daily contact plus HUAM group, a difference that was not significant. The incidence of preterm birth less than 35 weeks' gestation was 14% of the weekly contact group, 13% of the daily contact group, and 13% in the daily contact plus HUAM group. Similarly, the number of infants with birth weight less than 2500 g, mean days gained in utero, and neonatal outcomes were not statistically different between the three groups. This study, like that of the Collaborative Home Uterine Monitoring Study Group [55], failed to demonstrate a difference associated with the addition of HUAM to a protocol of frequent perinatal nursing contact, but again did not have a standard high-risk care group typical of what patients currently receive in clinical practice.

A prospective randomized trial was performed by Brown and colleagues [57] in 1999 focusing on women who had already undergone successful tocolysis for preterm labor. Following tocolysis, 86 women were randomized to an HUAM group and 80 were assigned to an unmonitored group. Both groups received daily telephone contact and oral terbutaline therapy. The HUAM group had a lower rate of preterm delivery less than 35 weeks' gestation (10.9% versus 15%) and fewer deliveries less than 37 weeks (48.8% in the HUAM group versus 60% in the unmonitored group). Unfortunately, the sample size was not large enough to demonstrate significance to these clinical differences. A power analysis performed by the authors indicated that they would have needed 438 women rather than the 162 they recruited to demonstrate a significant difference in the rate of preterm delivery less than 35 weeks' gestation. The control group also received daily nursing contact placing it outside a standard care protocol and making it more difficult to show a significant difference compared with the HUAM intervention. Although not significant, the HUAM group had an 11% lower rate of NICU admissions, a 25% lower rate of NICU days, and a 37% lower rate of mechanical ventilation.

Meta-analysis of home uterine activity monitor

The role of HUAM in preterm birth prevention has also been the subject of two meta-analyses, not surprisingly with conflicting results. In 1992 Grimes and Shulz [58] analyzed the five published randomized control trials of HUAM and found them all to have serious methodologic deficiencies. After ranking the strength of the methodologic approaches they concluded that four of the five trials demonstrated no significant benefit associated with HUAM. They found that the combined crude relative risk for all five studies was 0.9 and suggested that the small improvement in preterm birth rates was likely the result of the methodologic flaws. They concluded that the value of HUAM versus daily perinatal nursing contact was basically unproved. Also in 1992, Colton and colleagues [59] from the Boston University School of Public Health performed a meta-analysis of HUAM including the studies by Mou and colleagues [46] and Katz and colleagues [35,36], not reviewed by Grimes and Shultz [58]. In addition, they reviewed the studies by Dyson and colleagues [56] and Mou and colleagues [46] separately because of their methodologic superiority. Unpublished data were gathered from the authors of each of the trials to make them as similar as possible and overcome some of the methodologic deficiencies described in the Grimes and Shultz [58] meta-analysis. They found that HUAM was associated with an earlier diagnosis of preterm labor based on an increased percentage of women presenting in preterm labor with a cervical dilatation less than or equal to 2 cm. They found that HUAM was associated with a statistically significant reduction of 53% in the risk of preterm birth when the cervical dilatation was 2 cm or less ($P < .001$). Among all randomized women, in addition to a reduced frequency of preterm birth, they also found a higher mean birth weight and a lower frequency of NICU admission. Meta-analysis of the studies that controlled for nursing contact showed no difference or a stronger pooled effect compared with studies that did not control for this variable suggesting that the bias attributed to the nursing contact feature of HUAM is not as appreciable as some critics had suggested.

The most recent ACOG practice bulletin in 2001, "Assessment of Risk Factors for Preterm Birth," supplants its previous committee opinions regarding HUAM [60]. In that practice bulletin HUAM is discussed together with other screening tests, such as salivary estriol and bacterial vaginosis assessment. It concludes that the current data do not support the use of these modalities to identify or prevent preterm birth. That publication, however, includes much of the same data analysis present in its 1996 committee opinion. In that committee opinion, 10 randomized clinical trials were summarized, eight of which showed consistent benefit in terms of early diagnosis of preterm labor, a reduction in the preterm birth rate, and benefit to the neonate. The 1996 publication states that the evidence supports the hypothesis that the use of HUAM in pregnancies at high risk for preterm birth results in less cervical dilatation at the time of admission to the hospital for preterm labor, a position also supported by the FDA. The practice bulletin notes that in many of the studies the demonstrated benefit in reducing preterm birth occurred only in the women (compared with controls) who developed preterm labor. Many of the statistically significant differences between HUAM patients and controls became insignificant when the denominator was changed from the preterm labor patients to the entire randomized cohort.

Although this statistical criticism is valid from an "intent to treat" perspective it remains intuitive that it is those women who experience preterm labor where HUAM is likely to be of benefit and might serve to prevent adverse obstetric and neonatal outcomes. Further, follow-up evaluation of all randomized patients in the Mou and colleagues [46] trial and in the Wapner and colleagues [54] trial demonstrated clear improvement in obstetric and neonatal outcomes as does the meta-analysis performed by Colton and colleagues [59]. Ultimately, despite what seems to be overwhelming evidence, ACOG concludes that the data are insufficient to support a benefit for HUAM in preventing preterm birth.

Summary

The frustrating aspect of evidence-based medicine is that the evidence frequently generates more questions than it answers. The currently available basic and clinical data suggest that HUAM with or without perinatal nursing contact can reduce the risk of preterm birth and improve perinatal outcomes. Failures in the battle against preterm delivery probably arise from the more global failure to understand the complexities of prematurity and its treatment. There is a need to understand better the enigmatic and powerful forces that initiate the cascade of events leading to preterm labor and how to identify women experiencing that cascade. Better treatments are needed to interrupt the cascade, to arrest preterm labor, and prevent its recurrence. Finally, better measures of successful treatment are needed. The yardstick of delivery before or at term is too crude a parameter to measure successful obstetric interventions.

In the meantime, however, credit should be given to HUAM where credit is due. It accurately identifies prelabor uterine activity that is present throughout the latter half of gestation, usually below the threshold of patient self-detection. HUAM has the capability of making the diagnosis of preterm labor earlier than does the patient left to her own perceptive capabilities. This seems to be a consequence of an increase in mild to moderate uterine contraction frequency that occurs 24 to 28 hours before the patient-identified diagnosis of preterm labor. HUAM has been shown to reduce the risk of preterm birth, improve the gestational age at delivery, increase birth weight, and improve perinatal outcome in virtually every prospective randomized trial where the comparison group received standard high-risk obstetric care typified by preterm birth prevention education and instruction in the self-palpation of uterine activity. In no study has a surveillance program inclusive of HUAM been associated with an over-diagnosis of preterm labor. The benefits of HUAM, however, cannot be differentiated from other components of the surveillance program, specifically frequent perinatal nursing contact, improved patient access, and the increased rest associated with monitoring. In those studies that have failed to show a benefit associated with HUAM, the control group almost always includes some or all of these added surveillance elements that move the control group beyond the current standard of care for patients at risk for preterm birth.

The data are absolutely clear that HUAM and daily nursing contact are superior to routine care for the prevention of preterm birth. This was acknowledged by the ACOG committee opinion of more than a decade ago in 1992 [51]. Yet, despite global failure to reduce the rates of preterm birth in this country and the desperation to find an intervention that is effective in reducing this obstetric risk, very few practices have adopted increased prenatal surveillance using either frequent perinatal nursing contact or HUAM. It seems that preterm birth prevention is going to require a greater effort and cost than society has been willing to expend to date. It is possible that with improved techniques to identify those women at highest risk for preterm birth, with more successful therapies to interrupt the cascade of the preterm labor syndrome, or with better measures of tocolytic success, HUAM might be better recognized as a valuable adjunct to the obstetric management of this problem.

References

[1] Alvarez H, Caldeyro-Barcia R. Contractility of the human uterus recorded by new methods. Surg Gynecol Obstet 1950;91:1–11.
[2] Reynolds SRM, Harris JS, Kaiser IH. Clinical measurement of uterine forces in pregnancy and labor. Springfield (IL): Charles C Thomas; 1954.
[3] Moore TR, Iams JD, Creasy RK, et al. Diurnal and gestational patterns of uterine activity in normal human pregnancy. Obstet Gynecol 1994;83:517–23.
[4] Nageotte MP, Dorchester W, Porto M, et al. Quantification of uterine activity preceding preterm, term, and post-term labor. Am J Obstet Gynecol 1988;158:1254–9.
[5] Zahn V. Uterine contractions during pregnancy. J Perinat Med 1984;12:107–13.
[6] Araki R. The investigations of the effect of daily activity on the uterine contraction during pregnancy. Acta Obstet Gynecol Jpn 1984;36:589–93.
[7] Germain AM, Valenzuela GJ, Ivankovic M, et al. Relationship of circadian rhythms of uterine activity with term and preterm delivery. Am J Obstet Gynecol 1993;168:1271–6.
[8] Schwenzer TH, Schumann R, Halberstadt E. The importance of 24 hour cardiotocographic monitoring during tocolytic therapy. In: Jung H, Lambert J, editors. Beta-mimetic dugs in obstetrics and perinatology. New York: Thieme-Stratton; 1982. p. 60–4.
[9] Bruns PD, Taylor ES, Anker RM, et al. Uterine contractility, circulation and urinary steroids in premature delivery. Am J Obstet Gynecol 1957;71:579–88.
[10] Aubry RH, Pennington JC. Identification and evaluation of high risk pregnancy: the perinatal concept. Clin Obstet Gynecol 1973;16:3–13.
[11] Bell R. The prediction of preterm labor by recording spontaneous antenatal uterine activity. Br J Obstet Gynaecol 1983;90:884–9.
[12] Katz M, Gill PJ, Newman RB. Detection of preterm labor by ambulatory monitoring of uterine activity: a preliminary report. Obstet Gynecol 1986;68:773–89.
[13] Bentley DL, Bentley JL, Watson DL, et al. Relationship of uterine contractility to preterm labor. Obstet Gynecol 1990;76:36–8.
[14] Main DM, Katz M, Chiu G, et al. Intermittent weekly contraction monitoring to predict preterm labor in low risk women: a blinded study. Obstet Gynecol 1988;72:757–60.
[15] Newman RB, Gill PJ, Katz M. Uterine activity during pregnancy in ambulatory patients: comparison of singleton and twin gestations. Am J Obstet Gynecol 1986;154:530–1.
[16] Newman RB, Gill PJ, Campion S, et al. The influence of fetal number on antepartum uterine activity. Obstet Gynecol 1989;73:695–9.
[17] Warkentin B. Die uterin Aktivitat in der spatschwangerschaft. Z Geburtshilfe Perinatol 1976; 180:225–9.

[18] Creasy RK. Preterm labor and delivery. In: Creasy RK, Resnick R, editors. Maternal fetal medicine: principles and practice. Philadelphia: WB Saunders; 1984. p. 415–43.

[19] Newman RB, Gill PJ, Campion S, et al. Antepartum ambulatory tocodynamometry: the significance of low-amplitude, high-frequency contractions. Obstet Gynecol 1987;70:701–5.

[20] Kawarabayashi T, Kurayama K, Kishikawa T. Clinical features of small contraction wave recorded by an external tocodynamometer. Am J Obstet Gynecol 1988;158:474–8.

[21] Iams JD, Newman RB, Thom EA, et al. Frequency of uterine contractions and the risk of spontaneous preterm delivery. N Engl J Med 2002;346:250–5.

[22] Herron MA, Katz M, Creasy RK. Evaluation of a preterm birth preventive program: preliminary report. Obstet Gynecol 1982;59:452–6.

[23] Newman RB, Gill PJ, Wittreich P, et al. Maternal perception of prelabor uterine activity. Obstet Gynecol 1986;68:765–9.

[24] Newman RB, Campbell BA, Stramm SL. Objective tocodynamometry identifies labor onset earlier than subjective maternal perception. Obstet Gynecol 1990;75:1089–92.

[25] Beckmann CA, Beckmann CRB, Stanziano GJ, et al. Accuracy of maternal perception of preterm uterine activity. Am J Obstet Gynecol 1996;174:672–5.

[26] Martin RW, Gookin KS, Hill WC, et al. Uterine activity compared with symptomatology in the detection of preterm labor. Obstet Gynecol 1990;76:19–23.

[27] Iams JD, Johnson FF, Hamer C. Uterine activity and symptoms as predictors of preterm labor. Obstet Gynecol 1990;76:42–5.

[28] Dyson DC, Crites YM, Ray DA, et al. Prevention of preterm birth in high risk patients: the role of education and provider contact vs home uterine monitoring. Am J Obstet Gynecol 1991;164:756–62.

[29] Iams JD. A prospective evaluation of the signs and symptoms of preterm labor. Obstet Gynecol 1994;84:227–30.

[30] Merkatz RB, Merkatz IR. The contributions of the nurse and the machine in home uterine activity monitoring systems. Am J Obstet Gynecol 1991;164:1159–62.

[31] Smyth CN. The guard-ring tocodynamometer: absolute measurement of intra-amniotic pressure by a new instrument. J Obstet Gynaecol Br Commow 1957;64:59–64.

[32] Hess LW, McCaul JF, Perry KG, et al. Correlation of uterine activity using the term-guard monitor vs standard external tocodynamometry compared with the intra-uterine pressure catheter. Obstet Gynecol 1990;76:52–5.

[33] Dickinson JE, Godfrey M, Legge M, et al. A validation study of home uterine activity monitoring technology in Western Australia. Aust N Z J Obstet Gynecol 1997;37:454–8.

[34] Newman RB, Richmond GS, Winston YE, et al. Antepartum uterine activity characteristics differentiating true from threatened preterm labor. Obstet Gynecol 1990;76:39–41.

[35] Katz M, Newman RB, Gill PJ. Assessment of uterine activity in ambulatory patients at high risk for preterm labor and delivery. Am J Obstet Gynecol 1986;154:44–7.

[36] Katz M, Gill PJ, Newman RB. Detection of preterm labor by ambulatory monitoring of uterine activity for the management of oral tocolysis. Am J Obstet Gynecol 1986;154:1253–6.

[37] Morrison JC, Martin Jr JN, Martin RW, et al. Prevention of preterm birth by ambulatory assessment of uterine activity: a randomized study. Am J Obstet Gynecol 1987;156:536–43.

[38] Porto M, Nageotte MP, Hill O, et al. The role of home uterine activity monitoring in the prevention of preterm birth [abstract]. Presented at the Seventh Annual Meeting of the Society of Perinatal Obstetricians. Lake Buena Vista, FL, February 6, 1987.

[39] Iams JD, Johnson FF, O'Shaughnessy RW, et al. A prospective random trial of home uterine activity monitoring in pregnancies at increased risk of preterm labor. Am J Obstet Gynecol 1987; 157:638–43.

[40] Iam JD, Johnson FF, O'Shaughnessy RW. A prospective random trial of home uterine activity monitoring in pregnancies at increased risk of preterm labor. Part II. Am J Obstet Gynecol 1988; 159:595–603.

[41] Committee on Obstetric Practice. Home uterine activity monitoring. ACOG Committee Opinion #172. Washington: American College of Obstetricians and Gynecologists; 1989.

[42] Brown E. Home monitoring of uterine activity. Diagnostic and Therapeutic Technology Assessment Evaluation (DATTA). JAMA 1989;261:1–7.

[43] Hill WC, Fleming AD, Martin RW, et al. Home uterine activity monitoring is associated with a reduction in preterm birth. Obstet Gynecol 1990;76:13–8.

[44] Blondel B, Breart G, Berthous Y, et al. Home uterine activity monitoring in France: a randomized, controlled trial. Am J Obstet Gynecol 1992;167:424–9.

[45] Rhoads GG, McNellis DC, Kessel SS. Home monitoring of uterine contractility. Summary of a workshop sponsored by the National Institute of Child Health and Human Development and the Bureau of Maternal and Child Health and Resources Development, Bethesda, Maryland, March 29–30, 1989. Am J Obstet Gynecol 1991;165:2–6.

[46] Mou SM, Sunjerji SG, Gall S, et al. Multicenter randomized clinical trial of home uterine activity monitoring for detection of preterm labor. Am J Obstet Gynecol 1991;165:858–66.

[47] Corwin MJ, Mou SM, Sunjerji SG, et al. Multicenter randomized clinical trial of home uterine activity monitoring: pregnancy outcomes for all women randomized. Am J Obstet Gynecol 1996; 175:1281–5.

[48] Yin L. A response from the FDA. N Engl J Med 1991;325:1377.

[49] Knuppel RA, Lake MF, Watson DL, et al. Preventing preterm birth in twin gestation: home uterine activity monitoring and perinatal nursing support. Obstet Gynecol 1990;76:24–7.

[50] Nagey DA, Bailey-Jones C, Herman AA. Randomized comparison of home uterine activity monitoring and routine care in patients discharged after treatment for preterm labor. Obstet Gynecol 1993;82:319–23.

[51] Committee on Obstetrics Practice. Home uterine activity monitoring. ACOG Committee Opinion #172. Washington: American College of Obstetricians and Gynecologists; 1992.

[52] US Preventive Services Task Force. Home uterine activity monitoring for preterm labor: review article. JAMA 1993;270:371–6.

[53] McLean M, Walters WAW, Smith R. Prediction and early diagnosis of preterm labor: a critical review. Obstet Gynecol Surv 1993;48:209–25.

[54] Wapner RJ, Cotton DB, Artal R, et al. A randomized multicentered trial assessing a home uterine activity monitoring device used in the absence of daily nursing contact. Am J Obstet Gynecol 1995;172:1026–34.

[55] The Collaborative Home Uterine Monitoring Study (CHUMS) Group. A multicenter randomized controlled trial of home uterine monitoring: active vs sham devise. Am J Obstet Gynecol 1995; 173:1120–7.

[56] Dyson DC, Danbe KH, Bamber JA, et al. Monitoring women at risk for preterm labor. N Engl J Med 1998;338:15–9.

[57] Brown HL, Britton KA, Brizendine EJ, et al. A randomized comparison of home uterine activity monitoring in the outpatient management of women treated for preterm labor. Am J Obstet Gynecol 1999;180:798–805.

[58] Grimes DA, Schulz KF. Randomized controlled trial of home uterine activity monitoring: a review and critique. Obstet Gynecol 1992;79:137–42.

[59] Colton T, Kayne JL, Zhang Y, et al. A meta-analysis of home uterine activity monitoring. Am J Obstet Gynecol 1995;173:1499–505.

[60] Committee on Practice Bulletins. Assessment of risk factors for preterm birth. ACOG Practice Bulletin 2001;31L:98.

ELSEVIER
SAUNDERS

Obstet Gynecol Clin N Am
32 (2005) 369–381

OBSTETRICS AND
GYNECOLOGY
CLINICS
OF NORTH AMERICA

Biochemical Markers for the Prediction of Preterm Labor

John D. Yeast, MD, MSPH[a,b,]*, George Lu, MD[a,c]

[a]Department of Obstetrics and Gynecology, University of Missouri-Kansas City, 2301 Holmes,
Kansas City, MO 64108, USA
[b]Saint Luke's Hospital of Kansas City, OPC-II, 4401 Wornall Road, Kansas City, MO 64111, USA
[c]Obstetrix Medical Group of Kansas and Missouri, OPC-II, 4401 Wornall Road,
Kansas City, MO 64111, USA

Preterm delivery is the largest contributor to perinatal morbidity and mortality throughout the world. In the United States, nearly 1 in every 8 infants is born prematurely. Although a portion of these births are indicated preterm deliveries, the frequency of spontaneous preterm birth has remained largely constant over the past 50 years. In 2002, 12.1% of all births occurred before 37 weeks' gestational age. This represents an actual increase of 14% since 1990. Although part of the contribution to preterm delivery has been an increase in multifetal gestations because of assisted reproduction, the rate of preterm delivery among singleton pregnancies has risen from 9.7% in 1990 to 10.4% in 2002 [1]. In addition, over 65% of infant mortality occurs in preterm infants, nearly 19,000 deaths annually [2].

The preterm delivery contribution to adverse outcome is largely related to gestational age at delivery. Infants born at less than 32 weeks' gestation experience significantly more morbidity than those born later. Although numerous factors may help predict preterm delivery risk, the most consistent differences in the prematurity rates relate to race. Non-Hispanic whites have the lowest rate of preterm delivery and very low birthweight, whereas non-Hispanic blacks have nearly double the incidence of preterm and very low birthweight deliveries (Table 1).

---

* Corresponding author. Department of Obstetrics and Gynecology, University of Missouri-Kansas City, 2301 Holmes, Kansas City, MO 64108.
E-mail address: jyeast@saint-lukes.org (J.D. Yeast).

0889-8545/05/$ – see front matter © 2005 Elsevier Inc. All rights reserved.
doi:10.1016/j.ogc.2005.04.002   *obgyn.theclinics.com*

Table 1
2002 rate of preterm birth in the United States by race and Hispanic origin of mother

	White	Non-Hispanic black	Hispanic
Less than 32 wk GA	1.14	3.50	1.48
Less than 37 wk GA	9.07	15.98	10.63
Total preterm rate	9.07	15.98	10.63

Reported as percent of total deliveries for race.
Abbreviation: GA, gestational age.
Data from National Vital Statistics Reports 2003;52:10.

Preterm deliveries can be categorized into three general groups. About 25% can be considered indicated preterm deliveries, caused by either unstable maternal indications or nonreassuring fetal status. Preterm premature rupture of the membranes results in about 30% of preterm deliveries [3]. The remaining 40% to 50% result from spontaneous preterm labor. Although certain risk factors have been identified that may increase the risk of premature delivery [4], most cases occur in patients without clearly identifiable risk factors. As a result, many investigators have tried to recognize tools that might lead to early and correct identification of preterm labor, or risk of preterm delivery. A recent survey discovered over 30,076 citations on screening and diagnosis of preterm labor, with 19 different tests identified as potential screens for preterm birth [5]. Over the past decade, cervical length screening and various biochemical markers have been primarily investigated as potential predictive or diagnostic markers for preterm labor [6,7].

As of early 2005, only two tests have received approval by the Food and Drug Administration as markers for preterm labor: fetal fibronectin (Adeza Biomedical, Sunnyvale, California) and salivary estriol (Salest, Biex, Dublin, California) [8]. A number of other markers have also been studied and continue to be evaluated. This article reviews current information on biologic and biochemical markers for threatened or actual preterm labor.

Fetal fibronectin

Fetal fibronectin is a stable glycoprotein found in the interface between the maternal and fetal components of the choriodecidual junction [9]. It has a relatively high concentration within the extracellular makeup of this layer [10]. Fetal fibronectin has a role in establishing blastocyst implantation and maintaining the integrity of the choriodecidual interface [11]. Cervicovaginal secretions contain fetal fibronectin early in gestation, and then again just before term labor [12]. Concentrations are normally quite low in the second and early third trimester (Fig. 1).

The characteristics noted previously make fetal fibronectin a logical marker for threatened or actual preterm labor. The preclinical onset of preterm labor

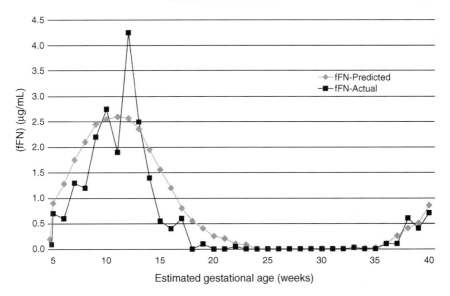

Fig. 1. Cervicovaginal fetal fibronectin levels during a normal pregnancy. Levels are normally elevated before 20 weeks' gestational age, and again near term. (*From* Ascarelli MH, Morrison JC. Use of fetal fibronectin in clinical practice. Obstet Gynecol Surv 1997;52:S1–12; with permission.)

seems to be associated with disruption of the choriodecidual junction, which in turn releases fetal fibronectin, which can be detected in the cervicovaginal mucous. Quantitation of fetal fibronectin can be performed and its presence or absence can then aid in the diagnosis and therapy of the patient. Initial clinical studies by Lockwood et al [9–11] indicated that fetal fibronectin was a sensitive marker for risk of preterm delivery, and was also a very significant tool when it was absent, because there seemed a very low risk of preterm labor occurring in the next few weeks.

Morrison et al [13] prospectively studied a small group of women who presented at 24 to 34 weeks' gestation with regular contractions, but a closed cervix. A fetal fibronectin sample was obtained, but the results were not available to the clinicians. In this study, all patients with a positive fetal fibronectin (N = 14) demonstrated preterm labor, and nine delivered preterm. In contrast, the remaining 14 women with a negative fetal fibronectin only developed preterm labor in four instances, and one patient delivered before 37 weeks' gestation. In this study, a positive fetal fibronectin yielded a sensitivity of 90% and a specificity of 72%. Of greatest significance was a negative fetal fibronectin, which demonstrated a 94% negative predictive value.

Iams et al [14], in a larger, multi-institutional study, also collected fetal fibronectin specimens from 192 women at 24 to 34 weeks' gestational age and presenting with regular uterine contractions. In this study, patients were eligible with cervical dilation up to 3 cm and intact membranes. In addition to risk of preterm delivery, this study compared fibronectin results with frequency of contractions and cervical dilation. In the study by Iams et al [14], fetal fibronectin was superior to both cervical dilation greater than 1 cm and contraction frequency in predicting preterm delivery. Fetal fibronectin assay was found to be most valuable at predicting preterm delivery within 7 days, with a sensitivity of 93% and specificity of 82% and negative predictive value of 99%.

Peaceman et al [15] published the largest study to date on the value of fetal fibronectin in the management of preterm labor. Over 700 patients were recruited from 10 different study centers. Specimen results were not available to clinicians providing care. The study demonstrated that a patient with a positive fetal fibronectin was more likely to deliver within 7 days (relative risk [RR] 25.9; 95% confidence interval [CI], 7.8–86), within 14 days (RR 20.4; 95% CI, 8.0–53), and before 37 weeks' gestational age (RR 2.9; 95% CI, 2.2–3.7). The authors also demonstrated with logistic regression analysis that a positive fetal fibronectin was a strong contributor to the risk of preterm delivery within 7 days. Multiple regression analysis similarly showed the presence of fetal fibronectin, use of tocolytic agents, prior preterm birth, and cervical dilation greater than 1 cm were all independently associated with birth before 37 weeks. A retrospective study by Lopez et al [16], using unblinded fetal fibronectin results, demonstrated a higher positive predictive value (40%) for delivery within 7 days than the study by Peaceman et al [15]. The sample size, however, was considerably smaller.

Lukes et al [17] reviewed predictors of positive fetal fibronectin from the study by Peaceman et al [15] to determine confounders contributing to the relatively low positive predictive value of the study. They found that there were five significant variables predicting a positive result: (1) uterine contractions, (2) cervical dilation, (3) sexual activity or cervical examination within 24 hours of specimen collection, and (5) vaginal bleeding. This study emphasized the importance of collecting the specimen before examining the cervix, to reduce the false-positive results.

Additional studies by Nageotte et al [18], Hellemans et al [19], and more recently by Garcia et al [20] and Sakai et al [21] demonstrated similar outcomes for the value of fetal fibronectin screening in patients at risk for preterm labor. Although several studies have reported the results of screening asymptomatic women, usually at the end of the second trimester, no study has shown any effective management tool to reduce the risk of preterm delivery. Goldenberg et al [22] reported the largest study to date of asymptomatic screening, but concluded it was not recommended because of lack of effective prevention and treatment.

Honest et al [23] conducted a meta-analysis of available studies on the use of fetal fibronectin sampling in women symptomatic for preterm contractions. The authors demonstrated that the sensitivity and positive predictive value of the test, although significant, remains low. The specificity and negative predictive value, however, are quite high. The sensitivity and positive predictive value of preterm birth before 37 weeks were 23% to 82% and 45% to 83%, respectively. Specificity and negative predictive values were 81% to 96% and 76% to 92%. The greatest clinical value of the test is excluding women with false labor from the costs and morbidity of aggressive treatment for preterm labor.

The clinical use of fetal fibronectin sampling was significantly improved with the introduction of a rapid, semiquantitative testing protocol, the Tli System (Adeza Biomedical, Sunnyvale, California). Before introduction of the Tli, analysis required specimen transportation to a central laboratory and ELISA testing. Results were not usually available until 24 to 36 hours postcollection. The Tli can be performed in a local hospital, and results are usually available in 1 to 2 hours. The Tli uses 50 ng/mL as a cutoff for reporting a positive result, as does the ELISA test.

Specimens for fetal fibronectin should be collected before digital examination, and preferably more than 24 hours since the last cervical examination or intercourse. Significant cervical dilation usually minimizes the value of the test, because treatment of preterm labor is warranted. Factors that can affect the result of the test other than those noted previously are premature rupture of membranes; vaginal bleeding (increased positives); the use of vaginal lubricants; and disinfectants (increased negatives).

There are now significant data to support the use of fetal fibronectin in evaluating preterm patients with symptomatic contractions and minimal cervical dilation. Although the positive predictive value of the test is low, a positive result does identify a group of patients that must be carefully watched for development of true preterm labor. Perhaps of greater significance, a negative result has a very high predictive value that the patient is not at risk of delivering prematurely, and can prevent unnecessary use of tocolytic agents and extended hospitalization.

Estriol

Contemporary interest in biologic markers, such as estrogen and cortisol, has evolved from studies conducted in a variety of animal species. Animal studies have shown that the fetus is responsible for the initiation of term and preterm labor through the activation of the fetal hypothalamic-pituitary-adrenal axis [24–26]. Rising levels of cortisol and estrogen are responsible for increasing the production of contraction-associated proteins, including myometrial receptors for oxytocin, and gap junctions between myometrial cells [27]. This "priming" effect enables the uterus to be more receptive to the stimulating effects of oxytocin and prostaglandins [28]. In the human placenta, however, the glucocorticoid-inducible enzyme 17α-hydroxylase–17,20-lyase that is crucial to such actions is absent [25]. The role of steroid hormones in human pregnancy seems to represent but one factor involved in the initiation of both preterm and term labor.

Estriol is the major form of circulating estrogen during pregnancy, the other forms being estrone and estradiol [29]. The levels of all three gradually increase throughout pregnancy, but there is an exponential rise in estriol levels after 34 weeks [29,30]. This surge in estriol level has been observed to occur 2 to 4 weeks before the onset of term labor [30], and its absence was noted among women who presented for induction at 42 weeks [31]. These early research efforts support the theories that estrogens, in particular estriol, are important in the initiation of labor in humans.

Measurements of estriol obtained from maternal saliva samples represent biologically active maternal serum levels, and have been used as a practical means for collecting samples [32,33]. The time of day, administration of corticosteroids, and dietary factors, however, seem to influence salivary estriol levels. A diurnal pattern has been observed, with higher levels occurring at night and lowest levels during the daytime [34,35]. Studies have shown that the administration of corticosteroids, including betamethasone, suppresses estriol levels [36,37] thereby potentially limiting the clinical use of this assay. There are also conflicting reports as to the effect of eating on estriol levels. Hull et al [34] noted decreased estriol levels after eating, which is contrary to those noted by the manufacturer of the assay (Biex product insert). Because of these potential interferences with the assay, the manufacturer has established guidelines for collection of the saliva sample to ensure reliable measurement of estriol.

There have been several published studies conducted to evaluate the ability of salivary estriol levels to predict preterm delivery in populations of asymptomatic women [38–40]. McGregor et al [34] prospectively evaluated serial salivary estriol levels in 241 women with varying risks for preterm delivery [38]. In women who delivered term and preterm, a gradual rise was noted in the highest weekly salivary estriol value. Consistent with prior studies was the observation of a surge in salivary estriol levels 3 weeks before delivery, whether the delivery was term or preterm. The investigators also noted that women with a resultant preterm delivery, when compared with those who delivered at term, consistently had higher weekly estriol levels between 24 and 34 weeks. Evaluation of the results from singleton pregnancies noted an estriol level of 2.3 ng/mL as the optimal cutoff for predicting those women at risk for preterm labor and delivery, with a sensitivity of 71%, specificity of 77%, and positive predictive value of 23%. When the test was applied retrospectively and compared with other clinical tools for predicting preterm delivery, salivary estriol was noted to be more accurate than conventional clinical risk factors (77% versus 37%, respectively).

In an extension of these findings, Heine et al [39,40] prospectively evaluated the predictive accuracy of salivary estriol with that of a modified Creasy score for predicting preterm labor and subsequent preterm delivery. A total of 956 women with singleton gestation were originally enrolled in the study between 21 and 25 weeks, among which 302 (31.6%) were categorized as high-risk with a Creasy score of at least 10 or more. In the analysis, 355 women (37%) were excluded because of a number of factors. Among the remaining 601 patients analyzed, there were 23 (3.8%) spontaneous preterm deliveries with 11 occurring in the high-risk group. In the high-risk group of women, the accuracy of a single positive salivary estriol test for predicting the pregnancy outcome was 68% versus 7% for the modified Creasy score. In a separate analysis [40], a single elevated salivary estriol level was significantly associated with a risk for preterm delivery with risk ratios between 3.4 and 4.2 in the general population, and in the individual high- and low-risk group. A second positive test within a week of the original positive test was associated with an increase in the risk for preterm delivery, with risk ratios of 5.8 to 8.5. Despite these strong associations, the ability of a positive result to predict the timing of preterm delivery was less robust. Only 23% of the women with a positive result delivered within a week of the test, whereas 54% delivered within 2 weeks and 85% delivered within 3 weeks of the test. A second positive result enhanced the predictive ability of the test, with 70% of women delivering within a week of the second result, 90% within 2 weeks, and 100% within 3 weeks. Although a single positive estriol test is associated with an increased risk of preterm delivery, it seems to be a better predictor of late (>34 weeks) preterm delivery. The clinical use of salivary estriol within the asymptomatic population is uncertain given its limited ability to predict preterm delivery proximate to a positive result and earlier preterm delivery (ie, those before 28 weeks), which contribute the greatest to the morbidity and mortality associated with preterm delivery.

The role of salivary estriol in women who present with symptomatic contractions or who have multiple gestations is unknown. Suppression of estriol by betamethasone and the uncertain effects of tocolytics on estriol levels represent a major hurdle in evaluating the use of this assay in women who present in preterm labor. In the study by McGregor et al [38], 26 women (10% of the study subjects) carried multiple gestations. These results were not included in the published data, however, and there have been no additional studies published to date evaluating the predictive value of salivary estriol in twin and triplet gestation. Additionally, the Food and Drug Administration approved salivary estriol assay has been approved for use only in women with singleton gestations. Because the current data suggest that salivary estriol levels are predictive of late preterm delivery (34–37 weeks) in singleton gestations, it is unlikely that such an assay is effective in predicting preterm delivery among women carrying twins, or higher-order pregnancies, because these populations are at substantial risk for early preterm delivery.

Corticotropin-releasing hormone

Corticotropin-releasing hormone (CRH) is expressed by the human placenta and the fetal membranes, with the highest level of production during the third trimester. This increase in production results in CRH being secreted into the fetal and maternal circulation. Unlike the usual inhibitory effects on CRH production, rising fetal cortisol levels during the third trimester stimulate the expression of CRH by the fetal membranes [24–28,41]. This paradoxical effect involving cortisol and placental CRH suggests that the placenta may be involved in the process of initiating labor, and has led some authors to propose the concept of a "placental clock" that determines the duration of the human pregnancy [41,42].

Initial studies yielded conflicting data as to the association between CRH and preterm delivery [43–45]. Berkowitz et al [43] retrospectively evaluated the CRH levels from frozen samples obtained during four gestational age intervals

(20–24 weeks, 24–28 weeks, 28–32 weeks, and 32–36 weeks). Of the 396 women evaluated, 45 (11%) were delivered preterm. There was no significant difference in the mean CRH among the women with a subsequent preterm birth compared with those who delivered at term. A sharp increase in CRH level was also noted with advancing gestational age, however, among all groups.

In contrast, Wadha et al [44,45] noted higher levels of CRH among those women who had a spontaneous preterm delivery. In the larger cohort study, CRH level were obtained at 33 weeks from 232 women with singleton pregnancies [45]. Delivery was preceded by labor in all women, with 22 (9.5%) women who delivered preterm (<37 weeks) and 18 (7.8%) who delivered postterm (>41 completed weeks). The CRH level at 33 weeks was significantly higher among women who delivered preterm when compared with those who delivered at term (215 $\pm$ 31.5 versus 139.6 $\pm$ 11.7 pg/mL [$\pm$ SEM], respectively; P <.01). Conversely, the CRH level of women who delivered postterm was significantly lower when compared with those who delivered at term (62 $\pm$ 11.4 versus 139.6 $\pm$ 11.7 pg/mL [$\pm$ SEM], respectively; P <.001). Women at high risk for preterm delivery were also noted to have higher CRH levels when compared with women at low risk (193.7 $\pm$ 22.3 versus 118.9 $\pm$ 10.9 pg/mL [$\pm$ SEM], respectively, P <.001). Even after adjusting for the potential confounding effect of clinical risk status for preterm delivery, an elevated CRH at 33 weeks was associated with a 3.3-fold increase in the RR for spontaneous preterm birth.

There have been several studies to determine the use of CRH for predicting subsequent preterm birth among women who present with threatened preterm labor [46–48]. Korebrits et al [46] evaluated 233 women who presented with preterm labor between 24 and 36 weeks with a singleton gestation. CRH levels were obtained at the time of admission, before the administration of any intervention. Maternal CRH was noted to be significantly higher among those who delivered within 24 hours admission (1343.3 $\pm$ 143.9 pg/mL, N = 81) when compared with those who delivered more than 24 hours later (714.5 $\pm$ 64.8 pg/mL, N = 144) and term control patients (445.3 $\pm$ 41 pg/mL, N = 28). When stratified by the gestational age at the time of presentation, these differences among the groups remained significant at 28 to 32 weeks and 32 to 36 weeks, but not in those presenting at 24 to 28 weeks.

Additional studies by Bisits et al [47] and Warren et al [48] have demonstrated similar trends in the CRH among those women who present with symptoms of preterm labor and subsequently deliver preterm. Despite these findings, the potential limitation of this particular assay in clinical practice was noted in the study by Warren et al [48]. In one subgroup of women, those who delivered preterm with clinical signs of infection had CRH levels that were comparable with normal pregnancies (660 $\pm$ 104 and 490 $\pm$ 50 pg/mL, respectively), and were significantly lower than those women who delivered preterm without signs of infection (1220 $\pm$ 170 pg/mL, P <.05) [48]. Additionally, they noted that the mean CRH level remained significantly elevated among those women who were treated for preterm labor and remained undelivered when compared with patients with a normal pregnancy. Such findings raise questions regarding the use of CRH for predicting early preterm delivery (<28 weeks), because such events are frequently associated with infection [49]. Furthermore, the clinical use of CRH is unknown among those women who present recurrent symptoms of preterm labor.

β-Human chorionic gonadotropin and alpha fetoprotein

Elevated levels of β-human chorionic gonadotropin (HCG) and alpha fetoprotein have been noted, either individually or in combination, to be associated with an increased risk for adverse pregnancy outcomes including preterm delivery [50–52]. Initial studies including those by Katz et al [50], Gonen et al [51], and Onderoglu and Kabukcu [52] noted the association between "unexplained" elevations of these maternal serum analytes, in women who had normal targeted ultrasound elevations to exclude spina bifida, and the subsequent risk of developing adverse pregnancy outcomes, including preterm delivery. They hypothesized that the increased levels in the maternal serum indicated either abnormal placentation or disruption in the integrity of the choriodecidual interface. Other studies confirmed such an association with measurement of these analytes in cervicovaginal specimens or from amniotic fluid samples [53,54]. In contrast, several studies challenged the association between abnormal HCG and alpha fetoprotein with adverse pregnancy outcomes [55,56].

Van Rijn et al [57] suggested that the discordance of the results among the studies was attributable to differences in the population being studied with regards to risk for preterm delivery. They evaluated the relationship between unexplained elevation of maternal serum HCG and alpha fetoprotein with the likelihood of various adverse pregnancy outcomes (including preterm delivery) in women at low and high risk for such events. Among the entire study population, the risk of preterm delivery before 34 weeks or any adverse pregnancy outcomes was increased (3.5, 2–6.3 and 3.1, 2.5–3.7, respectively; RR and 95% CI). When stratified by clinical risk status, the likelihood of any adverse pregnancy event among the women with any abnormal result was significantly increased in the low-risk group (3.8, 2–7; RR, 95% CI), but not in the high-risk group (1, 0.6–1.5; RR, 95% CI). Because of the size of the cohort, however, they could not compare specific outcomes, such as preterm delivery, between the low- and high-risk groups.

Despite the association between preterm delivery and HCG and alpha fetoprotein, the design of these earlier studies prevented any assessment with regards to the risk of preterm delivery. Gurbuz et al [58] prospectively evaluate 102 women who presented with symptoms of preterm labor and intact membranes. They noted a strong negative correlation between cervicovaginal HCG levels and the time from sampling until delivery ($R = -0.80$, $P < .0001$). At varying HCG cutoff values, they noted a robust ability to discriminate delivery in the near future. For example, the ability of an HCG greater than 32 mIU/mL to predict delivery within 7 days had positive and negative predictive values of 89% and

95%, respectively. These findings have yet to be confirmed by other investigators, but suggest a possible role for using HCG in the clinical setting.

Other biologic markers for predicting preterm labor

Several other biochemical markers have been associated with an increased risk of preterm delivery including activin, inhibin, and relaxin [59,60]. These glycoproteins are produced in the placenta and decidua and seem to facilitate the labor process through varying mechanisms: the former two through the release of local prostaglandins [61], whereas the latter seems to be involved in collagen remodeling within the amnion and chorion [60]. Although promising as potential markers, Plevyak et al [59] noted a significant effect with activin and inhibin levels only at 31 to 34 weeks' gestation. Further research is required to determine the clinical use of these markers for predicting preterm delivery.

Summary

Numerous markers continue to be studied as useful tools in the prevention of preterm delivery. Fetal fibronectin is the only assay widely used and consistently supported in recent studies. Although the predictive power of this marker is relatively low for preterm delivery, the specificity allows it to be used to exclude patients who would otherwise be aggressively treated for false preterm labor. It is possible that newer biochemical markers, either alone or in combination with existing markers, may be more sensitive in identifying patients truly at risk of preterm delivery.

References

[1] Sutton P, Mathews T. Trends in characteristics of births by state: United States, 1990, 1995, 2000–2002. Nat Vital Stat Reports 2004;52:2–152.
[2] Mathews T, Menecker F, MacDorman F. Infant mortality statistics from the 2002 period linked birth/infant death data set. Nat Vital Stat Reports 2004;53:1–32.
[3] Garite TM. Premature rupture of the membranes. In: Creasy RK, Resnik R, editors. Maternal fetal medicine. 5th edition. Philadelphia: WB Saunders; 2004. p. 723–39.
[4] Holbrook RH, Laros RK, Creasy RK. Evaluation of a risk-scoring system for prediction of preterm labor. Am J Perinatol 1989;6:62–8.
[5] Honest H, Bachmann LM, Khan K. Electronic searching of the literature for systematic reviews of screening and diagnostic tests for preterm birth. Eur J Obstet Gynecol Reprod Biol 2003; 107:19–23.
[6] Lockwood CJ, Dudenhausen JW. New approaches to the prediction of preterm delivery. J Perinat Med 1993;21:441–52.
[7] Goldenberg RL. The management of preterm labor. Obstet Gynecol 2002;100:1020–37.
[8] Ascarelli MH, Morrison JC. Use of fetal fibronectin in clinical practice. Obstet Gynecol Surv 1997;53:S1–12.

[9] Lockwood CJ, Wein R, Lapinski R, et al. The presence of cervical and vaginal fetal fibronectin predicts preterm delivery in an inner city obstetric population. Am J Obstet Gynecol 1993;169: 798–804.

[10] Lockwood CJ, Senyei AE, Dische MR, et al. Fetal fibronectin in cervical and vaginal secretions as a predictor of preterm delivery. N Engl J Med 1991;325:669–74.

[11] Feinberg RF, Kliman HJ, Lockwood CJ. Is oncofetal fibronectin a trophoblast blue for human implantation? Am J Pathol 1991;138:537–43.

[12] Yeast JD, Hickok D, Williams C. A positive fetal fibronectin test is associated with a reduced risk of failed induction. Obstet Gynecol 2004;103:70S.

[13] Morrison JC, Allbert JR, McLaughlin BN, et al. Oncofetal fibronectin in patients with false labor as a predictor of preterm delivery. Am J Obstet Gynecol 1993;168:538–42.

[14] Iams JD, Casal D, McGregor JA, et al. Fetal fibronectin improves the accuracy of diagnosis of preterm labor. Am J Obstet Gynecol 1995;173:141–5.

[15] Peaceman AM, Andrews WW, Thorp JM, et al. Fetal fibronectin as a predictor of preterm birth in patients with symptoms: a multicenter trial. Am J Obstet Gynecol 1997;177:13–8.

[16] Lopez RL, Francis JA, Garite TJ, et al. Fetal fibronectin detection as a predictor of preterm birth in actual clinical practice. Am J Obstet Gynecol 2000;182:1103–6.

[17] Lukes AS, Thorp JM, Eucker B, et al. Predictors of positivity for fetal fibronectin in patients with symptoms of preterm labor. Am J Obstet Gynecol 1997;176:639–41.

[18] Nageotte MP, Casal D, Senyei AF. Fetal fibronectin in patients at increased risk for premature birth. Am J Obstet Gynecol 1994;170:20–5.

[19] Hellemans P, Cerris I, Verdonk P. Fetal fibronectin detection for prediction of preterm birth in low risk women. Br J Obstet Gynaecol 1995;102:207–12.

[20] Garcia AA, Ayala-Mendez JA, Izquiredo-Puente JC, et al. Presence of fetal fibronectin in cervico-vaginal secretion as predictor of premature labor. Genecol Obstet Mex 1999;67:23–8.

[21] Sakai M, Sasaki Y, Yamagishi N, et al. The preterm labor index and fetal fibronectin for prediction of preterm delivery with intact membranes. Obstet Gynecol 2003;101:123–8.

[22] Goldenberg RL, Mercer BM, Meis PJ, et al. The Preterm Prediction Study: fetal fibronectin testing and spontaneous preterm birth. Obstet Gynecol 1996;87:643–8.

[23] Honest H, Bachmann LM, Gupta JK, et al. Accuracy of cervicovaginal fetal fibronectin test in predicting risk of spontaneous preterm birth: systematic review. BMJ 2002;325:1–10.

[24] Challis JRG, Gibb W. Control of parturition. Prenat Neonat Med 1996;1:283–91.

[25] Liggins GC. Initiation of labor. Biol Neonat 1989;55:366–75.

[26] Nathanielsz PW. Comparative studies on the initiation of labor. Eur J Obstet Gynecol Reprod Biol 1998;78:127–32.

[27] Garfield RE, Blennerhassett MG, Miller SM. Control of myometrial contractility: role and regulation of gap junctions. Oxf Rev Reprod Biol 1998;10:436–90.

[28] Norwitz ER, Robinson JN, Challis JRC. The control of labor. N Engl J Med 1999;341:660–6.

[29] Goodwin TM. A role for estriol in human labor, term and preterm. Am J Obstet Gynecol 1999; 180:S208–13.

[30] Darne J, McGarrigle HH, Lachelin GC. Saliva oestriol, oestradiol, oestrone and progesterone levels in pregnancy: spontaneous labour at term is preceded by a rise in salivary oestriol:progesterone ratio. Br J Obstet Gynaecol 1987;94:227–35.

[31] Moran DJ, McGarrigle HH, Lachelin GC. Lack of normal increase in saliva estriol/progesterone ratio in women with labor induced at 42 weeks' gestation. Am J Obstet Gynecol 1992;167: 1563–4.

[32] Vining RF, McGinley R, Rice BV. Saliva estriol measurements: an alternative to the assay of serum unconjugated estriol assessing feto-placental function. J Clin Endocrinol Metab 1983; 56:454–60.

[33] Voss HF. Saliva as a fluid for measurement of estriol levels. Am J Obstet Gynecol 1999; 180:226–31.

[34] Hull MG, Monro PP, Gilmer MD. Plasma unconjugated oestriol in late pregnancy: circadian variation and the effect of meals and a glucose load. Br J Obstet Gynaecol 1978;85:645–51.

[35] McGregor JA, Hastings C, Roberts T, et al. Diurnal variation in saliva estriol during pregnancy: a pilot study. Am J Obstet Gynecol 1999;180:S223–5.

[36] Hendershott CM, Dullien V, Goodwin TM. Serial betamethasone administration and the effect on maternal salivary estriol levels. J Soc Gynecol Invest 1996;3:276A.

[37] Leff RP, Goldkrand JW. The effect of betamethasone on salivary estriol. J Matern Fetal Neonatal Med 2002;11:192–5.

[38] McGregor JA, Jackson GM, Lachelin GC, et al. Salivary estriol as risk assessment for preterm labor: a prospective trial. Am J Obstet Gynecol 1995;173:1337–42.

[39] Heine RP, McGregor JA, Dullien VK. Accuracy of salivary estriol compared to traditional risk factor assessment in predicting preterm birth. Am J Obstet Gynecol 1999;180(1 Pt 3): S214–8.

[40] Heine RP, McGregor JA, Goodwin TM, et al. Serial salivary estriol to detect an increased risk of preterm birth. Obstet Gynecol 2000;96:490–7.

[41] Majzoub JA, McGregor JA, Lockwood CJ, et al. A central theory of preterm and term labor: putative role for corticotropin-releasing hormone. Am J Obstet Gynecol 1999;180:S232–41.

[42] McLean M, Bisits A, Davies J, et al. A placental clock controlling the length of human pregnancy. Nat Med 1995;1:460–3.

[43] Berkowitz GS, Lapinski RH, Lockwood CJ, et al. Corticotropin-releasing factor and its binding protein: maternal serum levels in term and preterm deliveries. Am J Obstet Gynecol 1996; 174:1477–83.

[44] Wadha PD, Porto M, Garite TJ, et al. Maternal corticotropin-releasing hormone levels in the early third trimester predict length of gestation in human pregnancy. Am J Obstet Gynecol 1998;179:1079–85.

[45] Wadha PD, Gartie TJ, Porto M, et al. Placental corticotropin-releasing hormone (CRH), spontaneous preterm birth, and fetal growth restriction: a prospective investigation. Am J Obstet Gynecol 2004;191:1063–9.

[46] Korebrits C, Ramirez MM, Watson L, et al. Maternal corticotrophin-releasing hormone is increased with impending preterm birth. J Clin Endocrinol Metab 1998;83:1585–91.

[47] Bisits A, Madsen G, McLean M, et al. Corticotropin-releasing hormone: a biochemical predictor of preterm delivery in a pilot randomized trial of the treatment of preterm labor. Am J Obstet Gynecol 1998;178:862–6.

[48] Warren WW, Patrick SL, Goland RS. Elevated maternal plasma corticotropin-releasing hormone levels in pregnancies complicated by preterm labor. Am J Obstet Gynecol 1992;166: 1198–207.

[49] Goldenberg RL, Hauth JC, Andrews WW. Intrauterine infection and preterm delivery. N Engl J Med 2000;342:1500–7.

[50] Katz VL, Chescheir NC, Cefalo RC. Unexplained elevations of maternal serum alpha-fetoprotein. Obstet Gynecol Surv 1990;45:719–26.

[51] Gonen R, Perez R, David M, et al. The association between unexplained second-trimester maternal serum HCG elevation and pregnancy complications. Obstet Gynecol 1992;80:83–6.

[52] Onderoglu LS, Kabukcu A. Elevated second trimester human chorionic gonadotropin level associated with adverse pregnancy outcome. Int J Gynecol Obstet 1997;56:245–9.

[53] Sanchez-Ramos L, Mentel C, Bertholf R, et al. Human chorionic gonadotropin in cervicovaginal secretions as a predictor of preterm delivery. Int J Gynaecol Obstet 2003;83:151–7.

[54] Wenstrom KD, Owen J, Davis RO, et al. Prognostic significance of unexplained elevated amniotic fluid alpha-fetoprotein. Obstet Gynecol 1996;87:213–6.

[55] Morssink LP, Kornman LH, Hallahan TW, et al. Maternal serum levels of free beta-HCG and PAPP-A in the first trimester of pregnancy are not associated with subsequent fetal growth retardation or preterm delivery. Prenat Diagn 1998;18:147–52.

[56] Verspyck E, Degre S, Hellot MF, et al. Amniotic fluid alpha-fetoprotein is not a useful biological marker of pregnancy outcome. Prenat Diagn 1999;19:1031–4.

[57] van Rijn M, van der Schouw YT, Hagenaars AM, et al. Adverse obstetric outcome in low- and high- risk pregnancies: predictive value of maternal serum screening. Obstet Gynecol 1999; 94:929–34.

[58] Gurbuz A, Karateke A, Ozturkmen M, et al. Human chorionic gonadotropin assay in cervical secretions for accurate diagnosis of preterm labor. Int J Gynaecol Obstet 2004;85:132 – 8.

[59] Plevyak MP, Lambert-Messerlian GM, Farina A, et al. Concentrations of serum total activin A and inhibin A in preterm and term labor patients: a cross-sectional study. J Soc Gynecol Investig 2003;10:231 – 6.

[60] Petersen LK, Skajaa K, Uldbjerg N. Serum relaxin as a potential marker for preterm labour. Br J Obstet Gynaecol 1992;92:292 – 5.

[61] Wallace EM, Healy DL. Inhibins and activins: roles in clinical practice. Br J Obstet Gynaecol 1996;103:945 – 56.

ELSEVIER
SAUNDERS

Obstet Gynecol Clin N Am
32 (2005) 383–396

OBSTETRICS AND
GYNECOLOGY
CLINICS
OF NORTH AMERICA

Cervical Sonography in Women with Symptoms of Preterm Labor

Vincenzo Berghella, MD[a],*, Amen Ness, MD[a],
George Bega, MD[a], Michele Berghella, MD[b]

[a]Division of Maternal-Fetal Medicine, Department of Obstetrics and Gynecology,
Jefferson Medical College of Thomas Jefferson University, 834 Chestnut Street, Suite 400,
Philadelphia, PA 19107, USA
[b]Department of Obstetrics and Gynecology, Ospedale 'SS Trinita' via Paolini, 28 Pescara, Italy

In the last few years, ultrasound of the cervix during pregnancy has been the focus of much research. Significant advances have been made in its technique and in understanding the proper role of this procedure in several clinical settings. This article reviews the evidence for the clinical role of transvaginal cervical assessment in women with symptoms of preterm labor (PTL).

Diagnosis of preterm labor and the limitations of manual cervical examination

The diagnosis of PTL is usually made between 20 and 36 weeks by regular contractions and cervical change detected by manual examination as dilation or effacement [1]. The standard assessment of women in PTL in most developed and underdeveloped nations includes only manual cervical assessment to document such cervical change. Manual cervical assessment is subjective and not very reproducible (interobserver variability of 52%) [2]. It is also not accurate for evaluating the internal os (the whole upper half of the cervix is not measurable by this method) [3]. This is a major shortcoming because in both term

* Corresponding author.
E-mail address: vincenzo.berghella@jefferson.edu (V. Berghella).

0889-8545/05/$ – see front matter © 2005 Elsevier Inc. All rights reserved.
doi:10.1016/j.ogc.2005.04.007

and PTL it is at the internal os (and not at the external os) that the cervix starts to shorten and dilate. Manual cervical assessment is also nonspecific, because about 15% of primiparous women and 17% to 35% of multiparous women who are delivered at term have cervices that are 1 to 2 cm dilated by manual examination in the late second trimester [4].

Although PTL precedes over 50% of preterm birth (PTB), less than 30% of all the women who present to the labor ward with signs or symptoms of PTL deliver before 35 weeks, and less than 10% deliver within 7 days [5,6]. The accurate diagnosis of PTL is an important goal, given that about 70% of patients in placebo-controlled tocolytic trials deliver at term (false-positives) and about 20% of patients sent home after evaluation of PTL deliver preterm (false-negatives) [7].

Transvaginal ultrasound versus digital examination of the cervix

Several studies [8–10] have compared the reliability, validity, and clinical use of digital examination with transvaginal ultrasound (TVU) for predicting PTB in women with the diagnosis of PTL. In all of these studies TVU was shown to be clearly superior to manual examination for evaluation of the cervix and prediction of PTB in women with PTL. The superiority of TVU is that it can detect shortening of the cervical canal before it becomes evident with manual examination [11]. TVU cervical length (CL) is clearly superior to the clinically used manual dilatation and effacement in prediction of PTB [12]. Other studies have confirmed the safety [13] and acceptability [14–17] of TVU of the cervix. No significant inoculation effect of bacteria was noted with TVU [13]. Only minimal or no discomfort was reported by women undergoing TVU, with pain or severe discomfort in less than 2% of women [15]. Over 99% of women agreed to have a similar procedure in the future [17]. Although the authors are not aware of a direct comparison of manual with TVU examinations, these safety and acceptability rates for TVU of the cervix compare well with manual examination rates.

Technique of cervical sonography

Transabdominal ultrasound of the cervix is inadequate because (1) fetal parts can obscure the cervix, especially after 20 weeks; (2) it requires bladder filling, which can elongate the cervix and mask funneling; and (3) the long distance from the probe to the cervix does not allow for clear visualization of the cervix. Because there are better techniques for assessment of the cervix, transabdominal ultrasound should not be used to assess the cervix in pregnancy.

Translabial (also known as transperineal) ultrasound is more useful. This technique involves having the woman lie on the table with the hips and knees flexed, while a gloved transducer is positioned on the perineum in a sagittal orientation between the patient's labia majora. This technique is not impaired by obstruction from fetal parts, and does not require bladder filling, achieving close to 100% visualization. Other advantages of this technique are (1) the transducer is closer to the cervix, but does not enter the vagina (so no pressure can be exerted on the cervix); (2) it does not require an additional transducer; and (3) it is well accepted by pregnant women. One drawback of this approach is that gas in the rectum can hamper visualization of the cervix, especially the external os. Another significant shortcoming is that this technique is difficult to master, probably because of the poor visualization usually achieved compared with TVU. Translabial ultrasound should only be used in the rare woman with PTL who declines TVU. The technique of TVU shares the advantages of translabial ultrasound, but the probe is even closer to the cervix, and the problem of obscuring bowel gas is eliminated. It has become the preferred, gold standard method of evaluating the cervix in clinical settings, including women with PTL.

The sonographer or physician should begin TVU of the cervix by having the woman empty her bladder. After preparing the clean probe covered by a condom the woman is asked to insert the probe in the introitus. At this point the sonographer or physician places the probe in the anterior fornix of the vagina, so to obtain a sagittal view of the cervix, with the long axis view of echogenic endocervical mucosa along the length of the canal. The probe is withdrawn slightly until the image is blurred, and enough pressure is then reapplied to restore the image (to avoid excessive pressure on the cervix, which can elongate it). It is important to enlarge the image so that the cervix occupies at least two thirds of the image, and external and internal os are well seen. At this point the CL is measured from the internal to the external os along the endocervical canal (Fig. 1). The authors now obtain at least three measurements, and record the shortest, best measurement in millimeters. CL may change over the 5- to 10-minute course of the TVU examination. It is important to use the best shortest

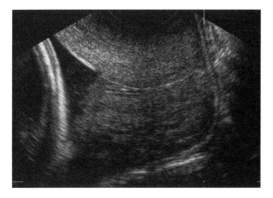

Fig. 1. Transvaginal ultrasound of cervix with normal (≥30 mm) cervical length.

CL for clinical management. Transfundal pressure does not add to the examination, and may not need to be performed [18].

For best results:

1. The internal os should be flat or at an isosceles angle with respect to the uterus and the external os should be visible and appear symmetric.
2. The whole length of the cervix should be visualized, so that the endocervical canal is visible from the internal to the external os.
3. A symmetric image of the external os should be obtained, so that the distance from the surface of the posterior lip to the cervical canal should be equal to the distance from the surface of the anterior lip to the cervical canal.
4. There should not be any increased echogenicity in the cervix (a sign of excessive pressure) [19].

Although TVU of the cervix is usually straightforward, there is some anatomic or technical difficulty encountered in about one fourth of patients [20].

1. Anatomic

Focal myometrial contraction: may obscure the internal os and make the cervix appear longer than it is.

Endocervical mucus or polyps: may appear to separate the anterior and posterior borders of the endocervical canal and make the cervix measure shorter than it is.

Rapid cervical change (dynamic cervix): CL may fluctuate during an examination. This is itself a risk factor for preterm delivery, especially if the shortest cervical measurement is below 15 mm.

2. Technical

Vaginal probe orientation: because the cervical canal has width (usually less than 1 cm in the axial plane) the manual examination may show a greater dilatation than the TVU CL in just the sagittal plane. In addition, in inexperienced hands, it is possible to obtain several diagonal angles through the cervix all giving a shorter CL than the true sagittal plane.

Pressure distortion: even minimal pressure on the cervix falsely elongates the CL measurement. Increased echogenicity within the cervix or just posterior to it usually indicates excessive probe pressure.

For these reasons, some have recommended that a sonographer be supervised for the first 50 procedures while expertise is being acquired.

Evaluation of patients with suspected preterm labor

TVU of the cervix has been studied extensively as a predictor of PTB in patients with symptoms of PTL (Table 1). Some studies evaluated CL on

Table 1
Prediction of PTB by TVU in women with symptoms of preterm labor (singleton pregnancies)

Author	N	PTB (%)	PTB defined (wk)	GA Studied (wk)	CL cutoff (mm)	% abn	Sens	Spec	PPV	NPV	RR
Murakawa [22]	32	34	N/A	25–35	<30	53	100	71	65	**100**	a
					<25	31	64	86	70	82	3.9
Iams [9][b]	60	40	<36	24–34	<30	73	100	44	55	**100**	a
Gomez [8]	59	37	<37	20–35	<18	41	73	78	67	83	3.9
					>0.52[c]	31	76	94	89	86	6.9
Timor-Trisch [25]	70	27	<37	20–35	Wedging	54	100	75	59	100	a
Rizzo [24]	108	44	<37	26–30	<20	N/A	68	79	71	76	3
Rozenberg [23]	76	26	<37	24–39	<26	39	75	73	50	89	4.6
Crane [10]	136	27	<37	23–33	<30	50	81	65	**46**	**90**	2.3
Venditelli [28][b]	200	41	<37	19–36	<30	64	83	88	54	**80**	2.8
Tekesin [30]	68	41	<37	20–35	<26	N/A	82	63	63	83	7.7[d]
Tsoi [5]	216	8	≤7 d	24–36	<15	20	94	89	37	99	101[d]
Fuchs [6]	253	8	≤7 d	24–35	<15	14	81	92	47	98	4

Author names in italics indicate studies of patients with PTL included in Leitich et al [21]. For studies
listing two sets of numbers for predictive accuracy, different CL cutoffs were used.
Abbreviations: % abn, percent abnormal; CL, cervical length; GA, gestational age; NPV, negative
predictive value; PPV, positive predictive value; PTB, preterm birth; PTB %, incidence of preterm
birth; sens, sensitivity; spec, specificity; TVU, transvaginal ultrasound.
  [a] Infinity, because one of the boxes was zero.
  [b] Twin pregnancies included.
  [c] Cervical index.
  [d] Odds ratio.

presentation, and some after interventions were already implemented to stop
the PTL. Although inclusion criteria for PTL and other variables in these studies were all slightly different, all showed a statistically significant predictive
accuracy of TVU for PTB. In 1999 Leitich and colleagues [21] performed a
systematic review of the use of TVU to predict PTB. They identified seven
studies that included women with preterm labor [8–10,22–25]. These studies
varied considerably in their population sizes, inclusion and outcome criteria, and
overall frequency of PTB; TVU CL was measured at a mean gestational age
between 28.6 and 31.1 weeks. Optimal cutoff value of CL for PTB also varied in
these studies from 18 to 30 mm. Nevertheless, the pooled data suggested a cutoff
of 30 mm has sufficient sensitivity to identify between 70% and 100% of women
who will have a PTB. Moreover, a CL of greater than 30 mm had a negative
predictive value close to 100% for PTB between 34 and 37 weeks, effectively
identifying patients who would not deliver preterm (see Table 1 italics). A cutoff
of about 20 mm had the best positive predictive value (70%). This information
may be helpful in avoiding hospitalization and more intensive therapies in
women who have a very low risk of PTB. Additional studies performed since this
review confirmed that TVU CL is a very good predictor of PTB in PTL patients.
These are also included in Table 1 (no italics).

What to measure when in preterm labor

CL is the most reproducible and valid variable for TVU cervical assessment in prediction of PTB (Fig. 2) [26]. The addition of funneling does not improve the prediction based on CL alone [27]. In women with PTL, funneling (>5 mm) was not found to be predictive of PTB, whereas CL was significantly predictive [28]. The addition of funneling information did not improve the predictive accuracy of TVU CL. In a large study of asymptomatic women, funneling predicted PTB and a short CL, but was more subjective, having a higher inter-observer variability [29]. All studies of TVU of the cervix in women with PTL except two mentioned CL as the best predictor of PTB in this population (see Table 1). Although one study reported cervical index (CL and funnel length) to be more predictive than CL alone [8], and another showed wedging (ie, funneling) to be as predictive as CL, most investigators have found measurement incorporating funnel length to be less reproducible and so less clinically useful.

A German group has shown that quantitative ultrasound gray-scale analysis is predictive of PTB in women with PTL [30]. In their study, this prediction was as good as CL, but the combination of the two did not improve the prediction of PTB based on CL alone. These results need to be replicated before being clinically useful. CL is all that needs to be measured on a TVU of the cervix for prediction of PTB in women with PTL.

When to measure transvaginal ultrasound cervical length in regards to contractions

Several studies have confirmed that CL changes during a contraction [31,32]. Dynamic cervical change detected by TVU is common in women with PTL symptoms, and is associated with uterine contractions. Asymptomatic women

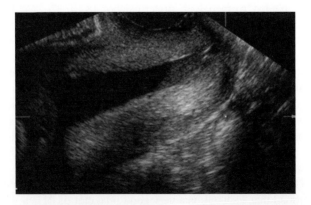

Fig. 2. Transvaginal ultrasound of cervix with short cervical length.

found to have a short CL often have contractions [33]. If women with a short CL are found to have contractions, their risk of PTB is double that of similar women without contractions [34]. In women with term labor, CL shortens about 50% on average during a contraction [31]. The degree of shortening is significantly greater in the normal latent and active phases compared with prolonged latent and active phases [31].

In general, the best predictive measurement of PTB in women with PTL is the shortest, best CL of multiple (at least three) measurements over the course of about 5 minutes. It is important to measure the CL over time because change may occur in about 50% of women with PTL over a 10-minute interval [32].

The possible use of repeat measurement of CL after tocolysis for PTL has been studied in 109 women [35]. These French authors confirmed that the initial CL at presentation with PTL predicts PTB. Although a repeat CL after 48 hours of successful tocolysis also predicted PTB, it was no better than the first measurement at presentation. Moreover, the variation in CL between first and repeat CL had a mean of only 3 mm, and was not predictive of PTB. After successful tocolysis, an increase of greater than or equal to 8 mm in CL compared with the initial CL was seen in 25% of women, whereas 25% of women had a decrease in CL. The increase in CL might be explained by relaxation of the upper cervix and lower uterine segment after the contractions stopped, but this is probably a temporary finding, because it was not predictive of PTB. They concluded that "to repeat ultrasonographic CL measurement after successful tocolysis is useless" [35].

It is important to emphasize that the shorter the CL, and the earlier the gestational age with a short CL, the higher the incidence of PTB. The clinician should also correlate the TVU CL information with the clinical situation. For example, for a given CL and gestational age, the incidence of PTB is very different based also on other risk factors, in particular multifetal gestations and prior PTB. Studies of predictive accuracy of CL that mix such populations (eg, singletons and twins) have poor clinical use (see Table 1).

Management of preterm labor and cervical sonography

Unfortunately, no prospective, randomized trial based on an intervention has been performed based on the association that short CL predicts PTB in women with PTL. Most research on PTL should have the goal of reducing PTB. There is a need to assess if the use of therapeutic interventions, such a bed rest, hospitalization, in utero transfer to a tertiary care center, tocolysis, and steroids, is improved by the use of TVU CL in this population. Additionally, there is a need to assess if the use of TVU CL helps clinicians better focus interventions for PTL, not only by intensifying treatment of high-risk PTL women, but also by decreasing or avoiding interventions in low-risk women. The effect of TVU CL on PTL management can be tested numerous ways. One approach is to randomize women in PTL to have the results of TVU CL available or not to the managing obstetrician. Such a study is underway at the authors' institution.

Evidence for clinical use of cervical sonography in women with preterm labor

Three nonrandomized trials have been reported on the effect of TVU CL on clinical management in women with PTL. Zalar [36] reported a decrease in incidence of birth weight less than 2500 g when TVU of the cervix was used to triage patients to bed rest and tocolysis, compared with historic controls. Rageth and colleagues [37], also using historic controls, limited tocolysis to patients with a CL of less than 30 mm. They demonstrated a decrease in the total number of hospitalization days, and the median length of hospitalization, without a change in the incidence of PTB. Among the 114 patients admitted for PTL, no patient with a CL greater than 30 mm delivered before 35 weeks. Most recently, a prospective, comparative study from Spain showed that in women with suspected PTL, assessing either the CL on admission or the lack of change in CL within 24 to 48 hours after admission reduced the mean duration of hospitalization by 2 days compared with controls in which the CL information was blinded [38]. Nevertheless, over 90% of all patients received tocolysis, and there was no difference in the frequency of PTB between the groups.

A cost-effectiveness analysis of the use of CL and fetal fibronectin (FFN) to guide treatment with tocolytics and steroids was performed by Mozurkewich and colleagues [39] comparing nine management options. Using the primary outcomes of respiratory distress and neonatal death, they found that universal administration of steroids, and using CL, FFN, or both to determine the need for hospitalization and tocolysis, resulted in the best balance of costs with the lowest risk of respiratory distress and neonatal death. Some units have stopped performing manual cervical assessments in women presenting with signs or symptoms or PTL, and instead use CL less than or equal to 26 mm together with at least two contractions per 10 minutes as criteria for admission and treatment [35]. Randomized trials should be performed in this area before clinical use can be recommended.

Preterm labor, short cervical length, and infection

In some women, PTL is a manifestation of intrauterine infection. The clinical diagnostic criteria for intrauterine infection have poor predictive value. There is a strong association between a short CL on TVU and infection. Recently, it has been shown that in women with symptoms of PTL, the shorter the CL, and the earlier the gestational age at PTL, the higher the incidence of amniocentesis-documented microbial invasion of the amniotic cavity [40]. Although routine amniocentesis in all women with symptoms of PTL may cause more harm than good, cervical sonography may help distinguish the subgroup of these women who are most at risk for intrauterine infection and indeed may warrant further infection work-up.

A short CL in women without symptoms of PTL may be caused by an intrinsic weakness of the cervix from traumatic or surgical damage; a congenital disorder; a connective tissue disease; or by premature cervical ripening, a process that is poorly understood but may be initiated by subclinical infection or inflammation [27]. A short CL may provide easier access of potentially pathologic vaginal organisms into the intrauterine environment, leading to prolonged subclinical chorioamnionitis and subsequent PTB. High amniotic fluid interleukin-6 (a proinflammatory cytokine), later development of chorioamnionitis, and acute inflammatory lesions of the placenta have all been associated with a short CL on TVU.

The role of fetal fibronectin with cervical sonography in women with preterm labor

In addition to TVU CL, FFN, a glycoprotein found in amniotic membranes, decidua, and cytotrophoblast, has been extensively studied and is widely accepted as a very good predictor of PTB. When FFN is present in cervicovaginal secretions after the 20th week of gestation, it predicts PTB better than cervical dilatation, effacement, and contraction frequency [9,41]. The first study to compare FFN with CL in women with PTL was performed by Rizzo and colleagues [24]. They noted improved predictive values adding CL to FFN. In their study, women with PTL and a positive FFN had a significantly shorter admission to delivery interval if they also had a short cervix less than 22 mm. Rozenberg and colleagues [23] showed that CL less than or equal to 26 mm and positive FFN ($\geq$50 ng/dL) were approximately equivalent in their prediction of PTB less than 37 weeks. They argued that for physicians equipped and trained to do reliable TVU of the cervix, the addition of FFN provided only slight benefits.

In 2002, Hincz and colleagues [42] proposed the "two-step test," sequentially combining sonographic CL with FFN. They demonstrated improved predictive values for admission-to-delivery interval with the combined use of FFN and CL for CL less than 30 mm but, because of small numbers of patients, only noted significance with CL in the 21 to 30 mm. As noted by others [9,22], no women had PTB if they had a CL greater than or equal to 31 mm upon presentation with PTL. Combining a highly sensitive test (identifying all those who will deliver early) with a highly specific test (identifying all those who will not deliver early) results in fewest false-positive and false-negative results. Using CL less than or equal to 31 (sensitivity approximately 100%) and FFN (specificity about 93%), few patients destined to deliver within 28 days would be missed, whereas patients who would not deliver within 28 days would be identified and could safely forego more intensive monitoring and therapy. It is important to recognize that in these studies the incidence of PTB varied considerably (26%–44%), the primary outcome varied from PTB less than 37 weeks to admission-to-delivery interval, and all patients were treated with tocolysis. These factors affect the generalizability and reliability of these studies, and should be taken into consideration when applying this information to other patient populations. For example, Iams and colleagues [43] calculated that the probability of PTB less than 35 weeks for asymptomatic women with a prior PTB, a CL greater than 35 mm, and a positive FFN was 28%, but the probability with same combination of results in women without a prior PTB was only 7%.

What if one suspects preterm premature rupture of membranes in the woman with preterm labor?

Four studies have examined the use of TVU of the cervix in patients with preterm premature rupture of membranes. Carlan and colleagues [44] demonstrated in a randomized trial the safety of performing TVU in this group. The incidence of chorioamnionitis, endometritis, and neonatal infection was the same in the 47 women with preterm premature rupture of membranes who had TVU and in the 45 women with preterm premature rupture of membranes who did not have TVU. In women between 24 and 34 weeks, they found that latency was 2 days shorter if the CL was less than or equal to 30 mm compared with CL greater than 30 mm (9 versus 11 days). Rizzo and colleagues [45] studied 92 women with preterm premature rupture of membranes between 24 and 32 weeks, and showed that a CL less than or equal to 20 mm was associated with a latency of 2 days (range 0–14) versus 6 days (range 0–36) if the CL was greater than 20 mm. Gire and colleagues [46] reported on 101 singleton pregnancies with preterm premature rupture of membranes at less than 34 weeks. A CL less than 20 mm was associated with a latency of 2.5 days versus 10 days if the CL was greater than or equal to 20 mm. Most recently Tsoi and colleagues [47] showed that TVU CL accurately predicts PTB within 7 days in women presenting with preterm premature rupture of membranes. These results should ensure the clinician that it is safe to perform CL by TVU in women with known or suspected preterm premature rupture of membranes because TVU is not associated with a significant inoculation effect [13]. TVU CL can be used to predict latency in all populations studied, including women with preterm premature rupture of membranes.

What if the woman with preterm labor is bleeding?

There are no specific studies to assess the safety of TVU of the cervix in women with PTL and vaginal bleeding. Studies in women with suspected placenta previa have shown that TVU is safe, and it is routinely recommended as an important diagnostic test in this clinical setting. The authors postulate that a properly performed TVU of the cervix is very safe for both mother and fetus in the pregnancy complicated by PTL and vaginal bleeding, and can add significant diagnostic information, which can improve management.

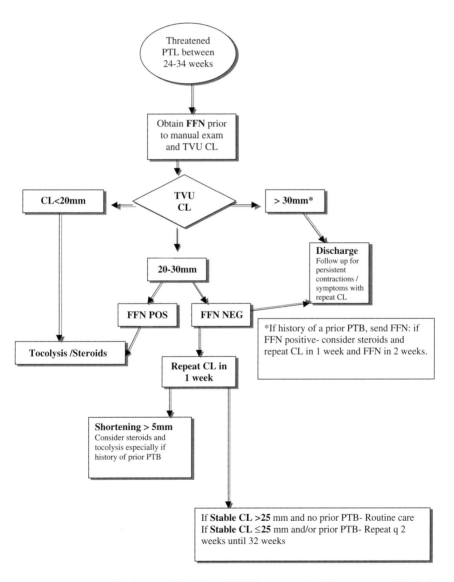

Fig. 3. Suggested algorithm for use of TVU CL and FFN in women with PTL symptoms. FFN, fetal fibronectin; NEG, negative; POS, positive; PTB, preterm birth; PTL, preterm labor; TVU CL, transvaginal ultrasound cervical length.

What if the woman in preterm labor has twins or a cerclage in place?

Unfortunately, there are no specific studies of women with PTL who are carrying multiple gestations or have a cerclage in place. In asymptomatic women with multifetal gestations or cerclage in place, TVU CL seems to be predictive of PTB [26].

Proposed management algorithm

Despite the absence of a randomized controlled study on which to base the management of PTL incorporating TVU CL, a suggested approach can be derived from the results of the currently available data (Fig. 3). It must be emphasized that this is one of many possible approaches, and is not supported by level A evidence. This approach uses the high sensitivity and negative predictive value of a CL of 30 mm, and the positive predictive value of a CL of 20 mm (highlighted in Table 1), and the specificity of FFN. It also recognizes that CL and FFN may identify different groups of patients at high risk for PTB, and that the predictive value of FFN and CL are dependent on the a priori risk of PTB in that population [43,48,49]. Because the symptoms of early PTL may be subtle and nonspecific, it is important, as noted by Iams [7], to be "liberal in looking for PTL, but conservative in diagnosis and treatment"; "the goal of first contact with a patient should be *sensitivity* while the goal of evaluation should be *specificity*" [7].

Summary

An ultrasound machine has been present in labor and delivery suites for decades for assessment of the fetus. It is time now to add a dedicated vaginal probe to this machine, for assessment of CL in women with PTL.

References

[1] Iams JD, Creasy RK. Preterm labor and delivery. In: Creasy RK, Resnik R, editors. Maternal-fetal medicine: principles and practice. 5th edition. Philadelphia: WB Saunders; 2004. p. 623–62.
[2] Phelps JY, Higby K, Smyth MH, et al. Accuracy and intraobserver variability of simulated cervical dilatation measurements. Am J Obstet Gynecol 1995;173:942–5.
[3] Michaels WH, Montgomery C, Karo J, et al. Ultrasound differentiation of the competent from the incompetent cervix: prevention of preterm delivery. Am J Obstet Gynecol 1986;154:537–46.
[4] Floyd WS. Cervical dilatation in the mid-trimester of pregnancy. Obstet Gynecol 1961;18: 380–1.
[5] Tsoi E, Akmal S, Rane S, et al. Ultrasound assessment of cervical length in threatened preterm labor. Ultrasound Obstet Gynecol 2003;21:552–5.
[6] Fuchs IB, Henrich W, Osthues K, et al. Sonographic cervical length in singleton pregnancies

with intact membranes presenting with threatened preterm labor. Ultrasound Obstet Gynecol 2004;24:554–7.

[7] Iams JD. Preterm birth. In: Gabbe SG, Niebyl JR, Simpson JL, editors. Obstetrics: normal and problem pregnancies. 4th edition. Philadelphia: Churchill Livingston; 2002. p. 755–826.

[8] Gomez R, Galasso M, Romero R, et al. Ultrasonographic examination of the uterine cervix is better than cervical digital examination as a predictor of the likelihood of premature delivery in patients with preterm labor and intact membranes. Am J Obstet Gynecol 1994;171:956–64.

[9] Iams JD, Paraskos J, Landon MB, et al. Cervical sonography in preterm labor. Obstet Gynecol 1994;84:40–6.

[10] Crane JMG, Van Den Hof M, Armson BA, et al. Transvaginal ultrasound in the prediction of preterm delivery: singleton and twin gestations. Obstet Gynecol 1997;90:357–63.

[11] Okitsu O, Miruma T, Nakayama T, et al. Early prediction of preterm delivery by transvaginal ultrasonography. Ultrasound Obstet Gynecol 1992;2:402–9.

[12] Berghella V, Tolosa JE, Kuhlman K, et al. Cervical ultrasonography compared with manual examination as a predictor of preterm delivery. Am J Obstet Gynecol 1997;177:723–30.

[13] Krebs-Jimenez J, Neubert AG. The microbiological effects of endovaginal sonographic assessment of cervical length. J Ultrasound Med 2002;21:727–9.

[14] Cowan Bennett C, Richards DS. Patient acceptance of endovaginal ultrasound. Ultrasound Obstet Gynecol 2000;15:52–5.

[15] Clement S, Candy B, Heath V, et al. Transvaginal ultrasound in pregnancy: its acceptability to women and maternal psychological morbidity. Ultrasound Obstet Gynecol 2003;22:508–14.

[16] Dutta RL, Economides DL. Patient acceptance of transvaginal sonography in the early pregnancy unit setting. Ultrasound Obstet Gynecol 2003;22:503–7.

[17] Braithwaite JM, Economides DL. Acceptability by patients of transvaginal sonography in the elective assessment of the first-trimester fetus. Ultrasound Obstet Gynecol 1997;9:91–3.

[18] Kurtzman JT, Jenkins SM, Brewster WR. Dynamic cervical change during real-time ultrasound: prospective characterization and comparison in patients with and without symptoms of preterm labor. Ultrasound Obstet Gynecol 2004;23:574–8.

[19] Burger M, Weber-Rossler T, Willmann M. measurement of the pregnant cervix by transvaginal sonography: an interobserver study and new standards to improve the interobserver variability. Ultrasound Obstet Gynecol 1997;9:188–93.

[20] Yost NP, Bloom SL, Twickler DM, et al. Pitfalls in ultrasonic cervical length measurement for predicting preterm birth. Obstet Gynecol 1999;93:510–6.

[21] Leitich H, Brunbauer M, Kaider A, et al. Cervical length and dilataion of the internal cervical os detected by vaginal ultrasonography as markers for preterm delivery: a systematic review. Am J Obstet Gynecol 1999;181:1465–72.

[22] Murakawa H, Utumi T, Hasegawa I, et al. Evaluation of threatened preterm delivery by transvaginal ultrasonographic measurement of cervical length. Obstet Gynecol 1993;82:829–32.

[23] Rozenberg P, Goffinet F, Malagrida L, et al. Evaluating the risk of preterm delivery: a comparison of fetal fibronectin and transvaginal ultrasonographic measurement of cervical length. Am J Obstet Gynecol 1997;176:196–9.

[24] Rizzo G, Capponi A, Arduini D, et al. The value of fetal fibronectin in cervical and vaginal secretions and of ultrasonographic examination of the uterine cervix in predicting premature delivery for patients with preterm labor and intact membranes. Am J Obstet Gynecol 1996; 175:1146–51.

[25] Timor-Tritsch IE, Boozarjomehri F, Masakowski MA, et al. Can a "snapshot" sagittal view of the cervix by transvaginal ultrasonography predict active preterm labor? Am J Obstet Gynecol 1996;174:990–5.

[26] Berghella V, Bega G, Tolosa JE, et al. Ultrasound assessment of the cervix. Clin Obstet Gynecol 2003;46:947–62.

[27] Owen J, Yost N, Berghella V, et al. Can shortened midtrimester cervical length predict very early spontaneous preterm birth? Am J Obstet Gynecol 2004;191:298–303.

[28] Vendittelli F, Mamelle N, Munoz F, et al. Transvaginal ultrasonography of the uterine cervix in hospitalized women with preterm labor. Int J Gynecol Obstet 2001;72:117–25.

[29] Iams JD, Goldenberg RL, Meis PJ, et al. The length of the cervix and the risk of spontaneous premature delivery. N Engl J Med 1996;334:567–72.

[30] Tekesin I, Hellmeyer L, Heller G, et al. Evaluation of quantitative ultrasound tissue characterization of the cervix and cervical length in the prediction of premature delivery for patients with spontaneous preterm labor. Am J Obstet Gynecol 2003;189:532–9.

[31] Saito M, Kozuma S, Kikuchi A, et al. Sonographic assessment of the cervix before, during and after a uterine contraction is effective in predicting the course of labor. Ultrasound Obstet Gynecol 2003;22:604–8.

[32] Kurtzman JT, Jenkins SM, Brewster WR. Dynamic cervical change during real-time ultrasound: prospective characterization and comparison in patients with and without symptoms of preterm labor. Ultrasound Obstet Gynecol 2004;23:574–8.

[33] Lewis D, Pelham J, Sawhney H, et al. Most asymptomatic pregnant women with a short cervix on ultrasound are having uterine contractions. Am J Obstet Gynecol 2001;185:S144.

[34] Berghella V, Iams JD, Newman RB, et al. Frequency of uterine contractions in asymptomatic pregnant women with or without a short cervix on transvaginal ultrasound. Am J Obstet Gynecol 2004;191:1253–6.

[35] Rozenberg P, Rudant J, Chevret S, et al. Repeat measurement of cervical length after successful tocolysis. Obstet Gynecol 2004;104:995–9.

[36] Zalar RW. Transvaginal ultrasound and preterm prelabor: a nonrandomized intervention study. Obstet Gynecol 1996;88:20–3.

[37] Rageth JC, Kernen B, Saurenmann E, et al. Premature contractions: possible influence of sonographic measurement of cervical length on clinical management. Ultrasound Obstet Gynecol 1997;9:183–7.

[38] Sanin-Blair J, Palachio M, Delgado J, et al. Impact of ultrasound cervical length assessment on duration of hospital stay in the clinical management of threatened preterm labor. Ultrasound Obstet Gynecol 2004;24:756–60.

[39] Mozurkewich E, Naglie G, Krahn M, et al. Predicting preterm birth: a cost-effectiveness analysis. Am J Obstet Gynecol 2000;182:1589–98.

[40] Gomez R, Romero R, Nien JK, et al. A short cervix in women with preterm labor and intact membranes: a risk factor for microbial invasion of the amniotic cavity. Obstet Gynecol 2005;192: 678–89.

[41] Peaceman AM, Andrews WW, Thorp JM, et al. Fetal fibronectin as a predictor of preterm birth in patients with symptoms: a multicenter trial. Obstet Gynecol 1997;177:13–8.

[42] Hincz P, Wilczynski J, Lozarzewski M, et al. Two-step test: the combined use of fetal fibronectin and sonographic examination of the uterine cervix for prediction of preterm delivery in symptomatic patients. Acta Obstet Gynecol Scand 2002;81:58–63.

[43] Iams JD, Goldenberg RL, Mercer BM, et al. The preterm prediction study: recurrence risk of spontaneous preterm birth. National Institute of Child Health and Human Development Maternal-Fetal Medicine Units Network. Am J Obstet Gynecol 1998;178:1035–40.

[44] Carlan SJ, Richmond LB, O'Brien WF. Randomized trail of endovaginal ultrasound in preterm premature rupture of membranes. Obstet Gynecol 1997;89:458–61.

[45] Rizzo G, Capponi A, Angeline E, et al. The value of transvaginal ultrasonographic examination of the uterine cervix in predicting preterm delivery in patients with preterm premature rupture of membranes. Ultrasound Obstet Gynecol 1998;11:23–9.

[46] Gire C, Faggianelli P, Nicaise C, et al. Ultrasonographic evaluation of cervical length in pregnancies complicated by preterm premature rupture of membranes. Ultrasound Obstet Gynecol 2002;19:565–9.

[47] Tsoi E, Fuchs I, Henrich W, et al. Sonographic measurement of cervical length in preterm prelabor amniorrhexis. Ultrasound Obstet Gynecol 2004;24:550–3.

[48] Goldenberg RL, Iams JD, Das A, et al. The Preterm Prediction Study: sequential cervical length and fetal fibronectin testing for the prediction of spontaneous preterm birth. Am J Obstet Gynecol 2000;182:636–43.

[49] Iams JD, Goldenberg RL, Mercer BM, et al. The preterm prediction study: can low-risk women destined for spontaneous preterm birth be identified? Am J Obstet Gynecol 2001;184:652–5.

ELSEVIER
SAUNDERS

Obstet Gynecol Clin N Am
32 (2005) 397–410

OBSTETRICS AND
GYNECOLOGY
CLINICS
OF NORTH AMERICA

Infection and Preterm Birth

Laura L. Klein, MD*, Ronald S. Gibbs, MD

*Department of Obstetrics and Gynecology, University of Colorado Health Sciences Center,
4200 East 9th Avenue, Box B-198, Denver, CO 80262, USA*

An estimated 50% of spontaneous preterm births are associated with ascending genital tract infection [1], and those occurring before 30 weeks' gestation are even more likely to be infection-related [2–4]. Because the earliest preterm births account for a disproportionate percentage of neonatal morbidity, infection-associated preterm birth represents an attractive area for intervention. Infections at multiple sites are associated with spontaneous preterm birth: (1) intrauterine infection, either overt or subclinical; (2) lower genital tract infection or colonization; and (3) distant infections, such as periodontitis. For each category of infection this article outlines the evidence for the association with preterm birth and suggests interventions to prolong pregnancy or prevent preterm birth.

Intrauterine infection and preterm birth

Early evidence for the contribution of intrauterine infection to preterm birth came from a pathologic study of over 7500 placentas [3]. Histologic evidence of chorioamnionitis (neutrophil infiltration of the fetal membranes) was found in 5% of all placentas but in 94% of the placentas of infants delivered at 21 to 24 weeks. The incidence of histologic chorioamnionitis was found to increase sequentially with decreasing gestational age. Most of these infections were subclinical because only 13.8% of women with placental histologic chorioamnionitis were febrile during labor [3]. This histologic study clearly demonstrated the association of inflammation with preterm birth but did not prove that all cases were caused by infection. More information was gleaned from a study by Hillier

---

* Corresponding author.
E-mail address: laura.klein@uchsc.edu (L.L. Klein).

doi:10.1016/j.ogc.2005.03.001
obgyn.theclinics.com

et al [5], which demonstrated that either histologic chorioamnionitis or the recovery of bacteria by culture of the placenta and fetal membranes was associated with preterm birth, but that the combination of the two was associated most strongly.

Studies evaluating amniotic fluid cultures in the setting of preterm labor with intact membranes have found a prevalence of intra-amniotic infection ranging from 0% to 24% [6]. This variability depends on several factors: (1) laboratory techniques, particularly whether or not specific cultures for genital mycoplasma are performed; (2) the definition of preterm labor, with more positive cultures in patients with advanced cervical dilation and women who actually deliver preterm [4]; and (3) the gestational age of the pregnancies studied [4,7]. The importance of culture techniques was illustrated in a study by Watts et al [2]: 40% of positive amniotic fluid cultures obtained in a research laboratory were missed by the clinical laboratory. In the setting of preterm labor with intact membranes, positive amniotic fluid cultures are associated with shorter intervals to delivery, failure of tocolysis, and increased neonatal morbidity [4,8,9]. Many infections are polymicrobial, and the most common organisms isolated are genital mycoplasma (*Ureaplasma urealyticum* and *Mycoplasma hominis*); anaerobes; group B streptococci; *Gardnerella vaginalis*; and gram-negative rods, including *Escherichia coli* [4,5,8].

By using more sensitive assays, such as polymerase chain reaction, bacteria can be detected in the amniotic fluid of 30% to 55% of patients in preterm labor [10–12]. The highest detection rates are found when sequences common to many different bacteria, such as portions of ribosomal RNA, are used as primers for polymerase chain reaction [10,12]. Primers specific to individual bacteria give more information on the exact organisms present [11]. Although polymerase chain reaction is very sensitive and rapid, the clinical significance of the presence of bacteria in the amniotic fluid by polymerase chain reaction remains unclear. Oyarzun et al [11] found that only 31% of patients with preterm labor and *E coli* detected in the amniotic fluid by polymerase chain reaction actually delivered before 37 weeks. This may indicate a benign low-level colonization rather than a clinically significant infection.

Neonatal consequences of intrauterine infection

The significance of intrauterine infection lies not only in its contribution to the overall problem of preterm birth, but also in its unique neonatal sequellae. In the short term, very-low-birthweight infants born to mothers with clinical chorioamnionitis have twofold to threefold higher rates of respiratory distress syndrome, sepsis, and seizures compared with infants of similar birthweight born to uninfected mothers [13]. Even preterm infants born to mothers with subclinical infection (positive amniocentesis cultures in the absence of fever or other clinical signs of infection) or inflammation (elevated amniotic fluid levels of tumor necrosis factor-α) have higher rates of death within 24 hours of birth, respiratory distress syndrome, intraventricular hemorrhage, necrotizing enterocolitis, and multiple organ dysfunction after adjustment for birthweight [7]. In the long term, preterm infants of mothers with clinical chorioamnionitis have a relative risk [RR] for cerebral palsy of 1.9, and for periventricular leukomalacia (the precursor lesion for cerebral palsy) of 3 [14,15].

Several studies have elegantly investigated how intrauterine infection leads to adverse neonatal outcomes. The determinant of fetal injury may be not only the presence of pathogenic bacteria but also the fetal response to intra-amniotic infection. It has become clear that this fetal response is implicated in both the initiation and perpetuation of the preterm labor process and in subsequent fetal injury. Among patients with preterm labor or preterm premature rupture of membranes (PPROM), the presence of a fetal inflammatory response, known as "fetal inflammatory response syndrome," defined by elevated fetal plasma interleukin-6, was associated with an odds ratio [OR] of 4.3 for severe neonatal morbidity (respiratory distress syndrome, sepsis, pneumonia, bronchopulmonary dysplasia, respiratory distress syndrome, periventricular leukomalacia, or necrotizing enterocolitis) after correction for gestational age and other variables [16]. In the setting of PPROM, an elevated fetal plasma interleukin-6 correlated strongly with spontaneous delivery within 48 and 72 hours, indicating that this fetal response may trigger preterm labor [17].

Similarly, fetal inflammatory response syndrome is postulated to lead to cerebral palsy by fetal overproduction of cytokines, which causes cerebral cellular damage [18]. Elevated amniotic fluid concentrations of tumor necrosis factor-α, interleukin-1β, and interleukin-6 correlate with the development of periventricular white matter lesions in preterm infants who deliver within 72 hours of amniocentesis [19]. Additionally, studies of the brains of preterm infants who died during the neonatal period have shown a strong correlation between expression of tumor necrosis factor-α, interleukin-1β, and interleukin-6 in infant brain tissue and periventricular leukomalacia [20].

Antibiotic treatment in patients with preterm labor

Based on the association between intrauterine infection and preterm birth outlined previously, it seems intuitive that antibiotics could be helpful in the treatment of preterm labor. Among patients in preterm labor with intact membranes, several studies have reported the effect of adjunctive use of antibiotics to prolong pregnancy. These studies have generally excluded women with any clinical evidence of chorioamnionitis and are aimed at the treatment of possible subclinical infection. One representative large trial (ORACLE II) demonstrated no improvement either in delaying delivery for 48 hours or in a composite outcome including neonatal death, chronic lung disease, or cerebral abnormality [21]. A recent meta-analysis from the Cochrane Library assessed 11 trials including 7428 women (ORACLE II dominated the analysis because of its size). As shown in Fig. 1, overall use of antibiotics did not decrease preterm birth, delivery within 48 hours, or perinatal mortality. The RR for neonatal death in the antibiotic group was 1.52 with the lower bound of the 95% confidence interval

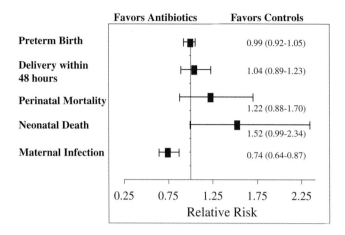

Fig. 1. Relative risks of adverse outcomes for any antibiotics versus no antibiotics for women in preterm labor with intact membranes. (*From* Klein LL, Gibbs RS. Use of microbial cultures and antibiotics in the prevention of infection-associated preterm birth. Am J Obstet Gynecol 2004;190: 1493–502; with permission.)

(CI) at 0.99 (just short of statistical significance). Maternal uterine infection was significantly reduced by use of antibiotics, but this benefit was not seen as a justification for widespread antibiotic use in preterm labor [22].

Because not all antibiotics are likely to have the same effect, this analysis also looked at the subgroup of trials using antibiotics "active against anaerobes," meaning either metronidazole or clindamycin. As shown in Fig. 2, in these three

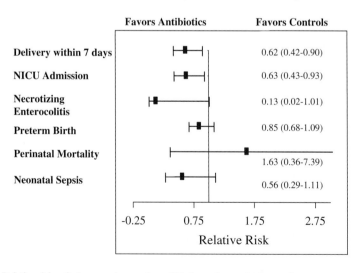

Fig. 2. Relative risks of adverse outcomes for antibiotics active against anaerobes versus no antibiotics for women in preterm labor with intact membranes. (*From* Klein LL, Gibbs RS. Use of microbial cultures and antibiotics in the prevention of infection-associated preterm birth. Am J Obstet Gynecol 2004;190:1493–502; with permission.)

trials use of antibiotics significantly reduced delivery within 7 days and NICU admission, but these benefits were not accompanied by significant reductions in the preterm birth rate, perinatal mortality, or neonatal sepsis. This analysis concluded that routine administration of antibiotics to women with preterm labor and intact membranes could not be recommended, because there were no clear improvements in neonatal outcomes and potentially a trend toward increased neonatal mortality [22]. Antibiotic use for prevention of perinatal group B streptococcal infection, however, is recommended [23].

Once intra-amniotic infection is definitively diagnosed, either by clinical criteria (fever, uterine tenderness, maternal or fetal tachycardia) or by amniocentesis, the standard of care is administration of intravenous antibiotics and delivery regardless of gestational age [24]. This strategy optimizes treatment of both maternal and fetal infection. Some have questioned whether administration of antibiotics to the mother could treat both maternal and fetal infection effectively while prolonging pregnancy. Several case reports have described eradication of bacteria from the amniotic fluid or reversal of clinical symptoms of chorioamnionitis with parenteral antibiotics, but no prospective trials have been performed and long-term outcomes have not been reported [25–28]. The concern is that if antibiotics do not adequately treat intrauterine infection, the fetus has prolonged exposure to both bacteria and inflammatory mediators with increased risk of long-term adverse outcomes. This concern is supported by strong evidence from a rabbit model of ascending intrauterine infection. Experiments with *E coli* have demonstrated that prompt intravenous administration of an antibiotic active against the infecting organism does not reliably prevent

---

Box 1. Antibiotics for patients in preterm labor: recommendations for clinical practice

- For patients in preterm labor with intact membranes, the prevalence of intra-amniotic infection is approximately 10% [4]. If any of the following criteria apply, the likelihood of infection is even higher and amniocentesis should be strongly considered:
    Any clinical signs or symptoms of chorioamnionitis
    Early gestational age (eg, ≤ 28 weeks)
    Failure of tocolysis (eg, before beginning a second tocolytic agent)
- Antibiotics should not be given routinely to patients in preterm labor with intact membranes for the purpose of prolonging pregnancy.
- Current Centers for Disease Control and Prevention guidelines should be followed regarding antibiotic administration for the prevention of perinatal group B streptococcal disease [23].

either intra-amniotic infection [29] or fetal brain white matter damage [30]. A key trial of antibiotic treatment for chorioamnionitis at term demonstrated improved neonatal outcomes with maternal antibiotic administration during labor compared with postpartum [31]. It is logical to assume that immediate antibiotic treatment with intravenous agents that cross the placenta well (eg, ampicillin and gentamicin) also improves outcomes for preterm infants.

Box 1 summarizes recommendations for clinical practice regarding intra-uterine infection in preterm labor.

Lower genital tract infections and preterm birth

The hypothesis that ascending lower genital tract infection leads to preterm labor has been supported by multiple in vivo and in vitro studies [32–34]. The entry of lower genital tract bacteria into the decidua is associated with recruitment of leukocytes followed by cytokine production [32]. Cytokines have been found to trigger prostaglandin synthesis in the amnion, chorion, decidua, and myometrium [32]. This, in turn, leads to uterine contractions, cervical dilatation, membrane exposure, and greater entry of microbes into the uterine cavity. Cytokines have also been found to stimulate production of matrix metalloproteinases by the chorion and amnion. Matrix metalloproteinases are implicated in both cervical ripening and degradation of the fetal membranes [32]. Lower genital tract bacteria may also act locally, producing enzymes, such as sialidase or mucinase, which may weaken protective cervical mucous and promote bacterial invasion of the upper genital tract [35]. The next sections outline the association between various antepartum infections and preterm birth, and the results of treatment trials for prevention of preterm birth.

Urinary tract infection

It has long been recognized that untreated pyelonephritis is associated with preterm labor. Closer investigation has revealed that even bacteriuria with no clinical symptoms of cystitis or pyelonephritis increases the risk of preterm birth. Women with untreated asymptomatic bacteriuria have a RR of 1.98 for preterm delivery [36]. Antibiotic treatment of asymptomatic bacteriuria reduces this risk by almost 50%, based on a meta-analysis of randomized placebo-controlled trials [36]. There is strong evidence to support screening and treatment for bacteriuria in all pregnant women at the first prenatal visit.

Cervicitis

Chlamydia trachomatis infection had not been consistently associated with an increased risk of preterm birth in older studies, which relied on culture for diagnosis [37,38]. It is now recognized, however, that DNA amplification techniques are more sensitive than culture for detection of chlamydial infection. The more recent Preterm Prediction Study used ligase chain reaction assay of urine specimens. Chlamydial infection detected at 24 weeks' gestation was found to be associated with double the risk of preterm birth, whereas infection detected at 28 weeks' gestation had no significant effect [39]. Unfortunately, randomized trials of treatment of *C trachomatis* during pregnancy have not demonstrated a consistent reduction in the rate of preterm birth [40]. Screening and treatment for *C trachomatis* in all pregnant women is recommended, however, to reduce vertical transmission and spread of sexually transmitted disease [41]. *Neisseria gonorrhoeae* infection has been associated with a 2.9-fold increased risk of preterm birth [42]. At-risk pregnant women should be screened and treated at the first prenatal visit to prevent vertical transmission and spread of sexually transmitted disease [41]. It is unknown whether treatment also reduces the risk of preterm birth.

Bacterial vaginosis

Bacterial vaginosis (BV) is associated with a twofold increased risk of preterm birth, with the greatest risk when BV is present before 16 weeks' gestation (OR = 7.55) [43]. This may indicate a critical period during early gestation when BV-related organisms can gain access to the upper genital tract and set the stage for preterm labor later in gestation. The results of treatment trials for pregnant women with BV have been heterogeneous, with anywhere from an 80% reduction to a twofold increase in preterm birth among women who received treatment [44]. The most recent Cochrane meta-analysis revealed no reduction in overall preterm birth with routine screening and treatment for BV. In women with a history of preterm birth, however, treatment was associated with a decrease in low birth weight and PPROM; the authors concluded that screening and treatment could be considered in this setting. Oral treatment was associated with a decrease in PPROM, whereas vaginal treatment had no effect [44]. A second meta-analysis by Leitich et al [45] analyzed subgroups based on risk for preterm birth and duration of treatment. There was no significant reduction in preterm delivery by treatment of all women with BV, women with BV and previous preterm birth, or women with BV at low risk for preterm birth. In the subset of women with both previous preterm birth and treatment for at least 7 days with an oral regimen, there was a highly significant reduction in preterm delivery (OR = 0.42, 95% CI, 0.27–0.67). In this meta-analysis there was no benefit accrued by vaginal treatment.

Since the publication of the Cochrane and Leitich meta-analyses, two additional prospective randomized trials have had intriguing results. In the first, by Lamont et al [46], treatment of low-risk women with BV with a 3-day course of intravaginal clindamycin cream resulted in a decreased incidence of preterm birth (4% versus 10%, $P < .03$). This trial differed from previous trials in that all patients were enrolled and treated before 20 weeks' gestation. In addition, patients had tests of cure performed with retreatment if BV persisted. A second trial treated low-risk women with BV between 12 and 22 weeks gestation with a 5-day course of oral clindamycin and again found a significant reduction in spontaneous preterm delivery (5% versus 12%) and late miscarriage (1% versus 4%) [47]. These trials suggest that early treatment of BV may be the key to prevention of preterm birth, but their results need to be replicated in high-risk populations, such as women with a prior preterm delivery.

An additional contributor to the relationship between BV and preterm birth may be genetics. A recent case-control study demonstrated that a variant in the promoter of the tumor necrosis factor-α gene in combination with BV carries a greatly increased risk of preterm birth, whereas either risk factor alone did not increase the preterm birth rate significantly [48,49]. This is an intriguing area for future research and could potentially lead to trials of treatment only for patients genetically predisposed to preterm birth.

Given the confusing evidence outlined previously, it is not surprising that the American College of Obstetricians and Gynecologists, the Centers for Disease Control and Prevention (CDC), the US Preventive Services Task Force, and the Cochrane reviewers differ in their recommendations for treatment of BV in pregnancy [41,44,50,51]. At the authors' institution, pregnant women with a history of preterm birth are screened at the first prenatal visit. They are treated with an oral agent (generally metronidazole) for 7 days based on the results of the Leitich meta-analysis, and tests of cure are generally performed with retreatment if needed.

Trichomoniasis

Trichomonas vaginalis infection has been associated with a small but significant increased risk of preterm birth (OR 1.3) [52]. Surprisingly, a large randomized clinical trial of screening and treatment for asymptomatic trichomoniasis found not merely the absence of benefit, but actually an increased risk of preterm birth (RR, 1.8, 95% CI, 1.2–2.7) [53]. A significant increase in low birth weight (RR, 2.49, 95% CI, 1.12–5.50) and a trend toward increased preterm birth and increased childhood mortality within the first 2 years of life were also noted in a recent randomized trial from Uganda [54]. The mechanism of the increase in preterm birth is unclear; one possible explanation is that dying trichomonads release either inflammatory mediators or viruses that trigger preterm labor [53]. Based on this concerning data it is clear that asymptomatic trichomoniasis should not be treated during pregnancy (eg, when it is found incidentally on a pap smear). These modest increases in preterm birth rates associated with treatment of trichomoniasis, however, do not justify withholding treatment from a symptomatic patient during pregnancy. The CDC's recommended treatment, oral metronidazole, has been shown to be safe even in the first trimester of pregnancy [55].

Other vaginal organisms

Vaginal colonization with *Candida*, group B streptococci, and *U urealyticum* has been studied and is not associated with increased risks of preterm birth [56–58]. Treatment for asymptomatic colonization with these organisms is not warranted. Group B streptococcal bacteriuria should be treated when detected, however, to prevent both symptomatic urinary tract infection and preterm birth. In addition, women with positive rectovaginal cultures for group B streptococci should receive intrapartum antibiotics to prevent neonatal infection per the CDC guidelines [23].

Fig. 3 summarizes the magnitude of the associations between several lower genital tract infections and preterm birth. Box 2 summarizes clinical recommendations for treatment of antepartum lower genital tract infection and colonization for the prevention of preterm birth.

Fetal fibronectin and intrauterine infection

Cervicovaginal fetal fibronectin, a basement membrane protein produced by the fetal membranes, is an established marker for an increased risk of preterm birth [59,60]. It has also been found to be associated with both clinical and histologic chorioamnionitis. It is hypothesized that early bacterial invasion of

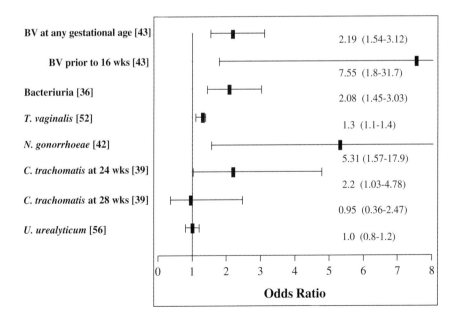

Fig. 3. Risks of preterm birth in women with selected lower genital tract organisms or bacterial vaginosis. Data are expressed as odds ratios and 95% confidence intervals. (*From* Klein LL, Gibbs RS. Use of microbial cultures and antibiotics in the prevention of infection-associated preterm birth. Am J Obstet Gynecol 2004;190:1493–502; with permission.)

**Box 2. Lower genital tract infections and prematurity:
recommendations for clinical practice**

- Bacteriuria: Screen and treat all patients at the first prenatal
  visit. Treatment of asymptomatic bacteriuria reduces preterm
  birth by close to 50%.
- *Chlamydia trachomatis*: Screen all patients using DNA amplification techniques with either cervical or urine specimens.
  Treatment does not seem to prevent preterm birth but does
  reduce vertical transmission and spread of sexually transmitted disease.
- *Neisseria gonorrhoeae*: Screen at-risk women at the first
  prenatal visit and treat per CDC guidelines to reduce vertical
  transmission and spread of sexually transmitted disease.
- Trichomoniasis: Do not screen asymptomatic patients because
  treatment may increase the risk of preterm birth. Symptomatic
  patients may be treated safely with oral metronidazole in
  any trimester.
- Bacterial vaginosis: Screen patients with a history of preterm
  birth. Treat with an oral agent for 7 days. Consider performing
  a test of cure with retreatment if needed.
- Group B streptococci: Do not treat positive rectovaginal
  cultures in the antepartum period. Follow the CDC guidelines
  regarding intrapartum antibiotics.

---

the chorioamnion causes inflammation with release of fetal fibronectin into the cervicovaginal secretions, and that this process eventually leads, at times several weeks later, to infection-related preterm labor [61]. A randomized trial of antibiotic treatment for asymptomatic patients with positive fetal fibronectin between 21 and 26 weeks' gestation was performed. Patients were treated with a 10-day course of metronidazole and erythromycin or placebo. There were no differences in the rates of preterm delivery between the antibiotic and placebo groups; and among a subgroup of women with a previous preterm birth, antibiotic treatment actually increased their risk of preterm birth [62]. Empiric antibiotic treatment cannot be recommended for women with positive fetal fibronectin tests.

Distant infections and preterm birth

Infections at sites distant from the uterus can potentially lead to preterm birth by hematogenous spread either of bacteria or cytokines. Periodontal disease is a common chronic inflammatory process involving gram-negative rods and anaerobes [63]. Severe or generalized periodontitis has recently been found to be associated with an increased risk of preterm birth, with an OR of 4.45 (95% CI, 2.16–9.18) for preterm delivery after adjusting for other known risk factors [64]. An initial American study of periodontal treatment during pregnancy suggested a trend toward a reduction in preterm birth [65]. In a larger study performed in Chile, 400 women with periodontal disease were randomized to periodontal treatment before 28 weeks' gestation versus postpartum. The prenatal treatment group had a significantly lower rate of preterm birth (1.84% versus 10.11%) [66]. This is an encouraging example of a simple intervention that may reduce the preterm birth rate.

Summary

Intrauterine infection is a major cause of preterm birth, and it also may have devastating neonatal consequences, such as cerebral palsy. A low threshold for using amniocentesis to diagnose intra-amniotic infection in the setting of preterm labor may improve neonatal outcome by allowing delivery before fulminant fetal infection develops. The routine use of antibiotics to prolong pregnancy once preterm labor has begun seems to be ineffective. This is likely the "too little too late" phenomena in that once the infectious-inflammatory cascade has reached the point of causing preterm labor it cannot be reversed.

In the antepartum period, treatment of bacteriuria, periodontal disease, and possibly BV is helpful in reducing the risk of preterm birth. Genetic susceptibility to infection-associated preterm birth is an intriguing area for further research. In the future clinicians may be able to tailor antibiotic therapy to the individual patient to prevent preterm birth more effectively.

References

[1] Lockwood CJ. Predicting premature delivery—no easy task. N Engl J Med 2002;346:282–4.
[2] Watts DH, Krohn MA, Hillier SL, et al. The association of occult amniotic fluid infection with gestational age and neonatal outcome among women in preterm labor. Obstet Gynecol 1992; 79:351–7.
[3] Russell P. Inflammatory lesions of the human placenta. I. Clinical significance of acute chorioamnionitis. Am J Diagn Gynecol Obstet 1979;1:127–37.
[4] Romero R, Sirtori M, Oyarzun E, et al. Infection and labor V. Prevalence, microbiology, and clinical significance of intraamniotic infection in women with preterm labor and intact membranes. Am J Obstet Gynecol 1989;161:817–24.
[5] Hillier SL, Krohn MA, Kiviat NB, et al. Microbiologic causes and neonatal outcomes associated with chorioamnion infection. Am J Obstet Gynecol 1991;165:955–61.
[6] Gibbs RS, Romero R, Hillier SL, et al. A review of premature birth and subclinical infection. Am J Obstet Gynecol 1992;166:1515–28.
[7] Hitti J, Tarczy-Hornoch P, Murphy J, et al. Amniotic fluid infection, cytokines, and adverse outcome among infants at 34 weeks' gestation or less. Obstet Gynecol 2001;98:1080–8.

[8] Romero R, Yoon BH, Mazor M, et al. The diagnostic and prognostic value of amniotic fluid white blood cell count, glucose, interleukin-6, and Gram stain in patients with preterm labor and intact membranes. Am J Obstet Gynecol 1993;169:805–16.

[9] Gravett MG, Hitti J, Hess DL, et al. Intrauterine infection and preterm delivery: evidence for activation of the fetal hypothalamic-pituitary-adrenal axis. Am J Obstet Gynecol 2000;182: 1404–13.

[10] Hitti J, Riley DE, Krohn MA, et al. Broad-spectrum bacterial rDNA polymerase chain reaction assay for detecting amniotic fluid infection among women in premature labor. Clin Infect Dis 1997;24:1228–32.

[11] Oyarzun E, Yamamoto M, Kato S, et al. Specific detection of 16 micro-organisms in amniotic fluid by polymerase chain reaction and its correlation with preterm delivery occurrence. Am J Obstet Gynecol 1998;179:1115–9.

[12] Markenson GR, Martin RK, Tillotson-Criss M, et al. The use of the polymerase chain reaction to detect bacteria in amniotic fluid in pregnancies complicated by preterm labor. Am J Obstet Gynecol 1997;177:1471–7.

[13] Alexander JM, Gilstrap LC, Cox SM, et al. Clinical chorioamnionitis and the prognosis for very low birth weight infants. Obstet Gynecol 1998;91:725–9.

[14] Wu YW, Colford Jr JM. Chorioamnionitis as a risk factor for cerebral palsy: a meta-analysis. JAMA 2000;284:1417–24.

[15] Leviton A, Paneth N. White matter damage in preterm newborns—an epidemiologic perspective. Early Hum Dev 1990;24:1–22.

[16] Gomez R, Romero R, Ghezzi F, et al. The fetal inflammatory response syndrome. Am J Obstet Gynecol 1998;179:194–202.

[17] Romero R, Gomez R, Ghezzi F, et al. A fetal systemic inflammatory response is followed by the spontaneous onset of preterm parturition. Am J Obstet Gynecol 1998;179:186–93.

[18] American College of Obstetricians and Gynecologists' Task Force on Neonatal encephalopathy and cerebral palsy. Washington: American Academy of Pediatrics; 2003.

[19] Yoon BH, Jun JK, Romero R, et al. Amniotic fluid inflammatory cytokines (interleukin-6, interleukin-1β, and tumor necrosis factor-α), neonatal brain white matter lesions, and cerebral palsy. Am J Obstet Gynecol 1997;177:19–26.

[20] Yoon BH, Romero R, Kim CJ, et al. High expression of tumor necrosis factor-alpha and interleukin-6 in periventricular leukomalacia. Am J Obstet Gynecol 1997;177:406–11.

[21] Kenyon SL, Taylor DJ, Tarnow-Mordi W, et al. Broad-spectrum antibiotics for spontaneous preterm labour: the ORACLE II randomised trial. Lancet 2001;357:989–94.

[22] King J, Flenady V. Prophylactic antibiotics for inhibiting preterm labour with intact membranes. The Cochrane Database of Systematic Reviews, vol. 1; 2003.

[23] Centers for Disease Control and Prevention. Prevention of perinatal group B streptococcal disease. Morbidity and Mortality Weekly Review 2002;51(RR-11):1–22.

[24] Gibbs RS, Sweet RL, Duff WP. Maternal and fetal infectious disorders. In: Creasy RK, Resnik R, editors. Maternal-fetal medicine. 5th edition. Philadelphia: WB Saunders; 2004. p. 741–801.

[25] Romero R, Scioscia AL, Edberg SC, et al. Use of parenteral antibiotic therapy to eradicate bacterial colonization of amniotic fluid in premature rupture of membranes. Obstet Gynecol 1986;67:15S–7S.

[26] Romero R, Hagay Z, Nores J, et al. Eradication of Ureaplasma urealyticum from the amniotic fluid with transplacental antibiotic treatment. Am J Obstet Gynecol 1992;166:618–20.

[27] Mazor M, Chaim W, Hershkowitz R, et al. Eradication of Viridans streptococci from the amniotic cavity with transplacental antibiotic treatment. Arch Gynecol Obstet 1994;255:147–51.

[28] Bollen B, Padwick M. Delayed delivery of second twin after chorioamnionitis and abortion of first twin at 21 weeks gestation. Eur J Obstet Gynecol Reprod Biol 2000;93:109–10.

[29] Gibbs RS, Davies JK, McDuffie RS, et al. Chronic intrauterine infection and inflammation in the preterm rabbit, despite antibiotic therapy. Am J Obstet Gynecol 2002;186:234–9.

[30] Debillon T, Gras-Leguen C, Verielle V, et al. Intrauterine infection induces programmed cell death in rabbit periventricular white matter. Pediatr Res 2000;47:736–42.

[31] Gibbs RS, Dinsmoor MJ, Newton ER, et al. A randomized trial of intrapartum versus immediate postpartum treatment of women with intra-amniotic infection. Obstet Gynecol 1988;72:
823–8.

[32] Keelan JA, Blumenstein M, Helliwell RJA, et al. Cytokines, prostaglandins and parturition—
a review. Placenta 2003;17:S33–46.

[33] Romero R, Espinoza J, Chaiworapongsa T, et al. Infection and prematurity and the role of
preventive strategies. Semin Neonatol 2002;7:259–74.

[34] Goldenberg RL, Hauth JC, Andrews WW. Intrauterine infection and preterm delivery. N Engl
J Med 2000;342:1500–7.

[35] McGregor JA, French JI, Jones W, et al. Bacterial vaginosis is associated with prematurity
and vaginal fluid mucinase and sialidase: results of a controlled trial of topical clindamycin
cream. Am J Obstet Gynecol 1994;170:1048–60.

[36] Romero R, Oyarzun E, Mazor M, et al. Meta-analysis of the relationship between asymptomatic bacteriuria and preterm delivery/low birth weight. Obstet Gynecol 1989;73:576–82.

[37] Harrison HR, Alexander ER, Weinstein L, et al. Cervical Chlamydia trachomatis and
mycoplasmal infections in pregnancy. JAMA 1983;250:1721–7.

[38] Sweet RL, Landers DV, Walker C, et al. Chlamydia trachomatis infection and pregnancy
outcome. Am J Obstet Gynecol 1987;156:824–31.

[39] Andrews WW, Goldenberg RL, Mercer B, et al. The Preterm Prediction Study: association of
second-trimester genitourinary chlamydial infection with subsequent spontaneous preterm birth.
Am J Obstet Gynecol 2000;183:662–8.

[40] Martin DH, Eschenbach DA, Cotch MF, et al. Double-blind placebo-controlled treatment trial
of Chlamydia trachomatis endocervical infections in pregnant women. Infect Dis Obstet
Gynecol 1997;5:10–7.

[41] Centers for Disease Control and Prevention. Sexually transmitted diseases treatment guidelines
2002. Morbidity and Mortality Weekly Review 2002;51(RR-6).

[42] Elliott B, Brunham RC, Laga M, et al. Maternal gonococcal infection as a preventable risk
factor for low birth weight. J Infect Dis 1990;161:531–6.

[43] Leitich H, Bodner-Adler B, Brunbauer M, et al. Bacterial vaginosis as a risk factor for preterm
delivery: a meta-analysis. Am J Obstet Gynecol 2003;189:139–47.

[44] McDonald H, Brocklehurst P, Parsons J, et al. Antibiotics for treating bacterial vaginosis in
pregnancy. The Cochrane Database of Systematic Reviews, vol. 1; 2003.

[45] Leitich H, Brunbauer M, Bodner-Adler B, et al. Antibiotic treatment of bacterial vaginosis in
pregnancy: a meta-analysis. Am J Obstet Gynecol 2003;188:752–8.

[46] Lamont RF, Duncan SLB, Mandal D, et al. Intravaginal clindamycin cream to reduce preterm
birth in women with abnormal genital tract flora. Obstet Gynecol 2003;101:516–22.

[47] Ugwumadu A, Manyonda I, Reid F, et al. Effect of early oral clindamycin on late miscarriage
and preterm delivery in asymptomatic women with abnormal vaginal flora and bacterial
vaginosis: a randomised controlled trial. Lancet 2003;361:983–8.

[48] Macones GA, Parry S, Elkousy M, et al. A polymorphism in the promoter region of TNF
and bacterial vaginosis: preliminary evidence of gene-environment interaction in the etiology
of spontaneous preterm birth. Am J Obstet Gynecol 2004;190:1504–8.

[49] Romero R, Chaiworapongsa T, Kuivaniemi H, et al. Bacterial vaginosis, the inflammatory
response and the risk of preterm birth: a role for genetic epidemiology in the prevention of
preterm birth. Am J Obstet Gynecol 2004;190:1509–19.

[50] American College of Obstetricians and Gynecologists. Assessment of risk factors for preterm
birth. Washington: ACOG Practice Bulletin no. 31; 2001.

[51] Guise JM, Mahon SM, Aickin M, et al. Screening for bacterial vaginosis in pregnancy. Am J
Prev Med 2001;20:62–72.

[52] Cotch MF, Pastorek JG, Nugent RP, et al. Trichomonas vaginalis associated with low birth
weight and preterm delivery. Sex Transm Dis 1997;24:353–60.

[53] Klebanoff MA, Carey JC, Hauth JC, et al. Failure of metronidazole to prevent preterm delivery
among pregnant women with asymptomatic Trichomonas vaginalis infection. N Engl J Med
2001;345:487–93.

[54] Kigozi GG, Brahmbhatt H, Wabwire-Mangen F, et al. Treatment of *Trichomonas* in pregnancy and adverse outcomes of pregnancy: a subanalysis of a randomized trial in Rakai, Uganda. Am J Obstet Gynecol 2003;189:1398–400.

[55] Burtin P, Taddio A, Ariburnu O, et al. Fetus-placenta-newborn: safety of metronidazole in pregnancy: a meta-analysis. Am J Obstet Gynecol 1995;172:525–9.

[56] Carey JC, Blackwelder WC, Nugent RP, et al. Antepartum cultures for *Ureaplasma urealyticum* are not useful in predicting pregnancy outcome. Am J Obstet Gynecol 1991;164:728–33.

[57] Cotch MF, Hillier SL, Gibbs RS, et al. Epidemiology and outcomes associated with moderate to heavy *Candida* colonization during pregnancy. Am J Obstet Gynecol 1998;178:374–80.

[58] Klebanoff MA, Regan JA, Rao AV, et al. Obstetrics: outcome of the vaginal infections and prematurity study: results of a clinical trial of erythromycin among pregnant women colonized with group B streptococci. Am J Obstet Gynecol 1995;172:1540–5.

[59] Goldenberg RL, Mercer BM, Meis PJ, et al. The preterm prediction study: fetal fibronectin testing and spontaneous preterm birth. Obstet Gynecol 1996;87:643–8.

[60] Goldenberg RL, Klebanoff M, Carey JC, et al. Vaginal fetal fibronectin measurements from 8 to 22 weeks' gestation and subsequent spontaneous preterm birth. Am J Obstet Gynecol 2000; 183:469–75.

[61] Goldenberg RL, Thom E, Moawad AH, et al. The preterm prediction study: fetal fibronectin, bacterial vaginosis, and peripartum infection. Obstet Gynecol 1996;87:656–60.

[62] Andrews WW, Sibai BH, Thom EA, et al. Randomized clinical trial of metronidazole plus erythromycin to prevent spontaneous preterm delivery in fetal fibronectin-positive women. Obstet Gynecol 2003;101:847–55.

[63] Jeffcoat MK, Geurs NC, Reddy MS, et al. Current evidence regarding periodontal disease as a risk factor for preterm birth. Ann Periodontol 2001;6:183–8.

[64] Jeffcoat MK, Geurs NC, Reddy MS, et al. Periodontal infection and preterm birth: results of a prospective study. J Am Dent Assoc 2001;132:875–80.

[65] Jeffcoat MK, Hauth JC, Geurs NC, et al. Periodontal disease and preterm birth: results of a pilot intervention study. J Periodontol 2003;74:1214–8.

[66] Lopez NJ, Smith PC, Gutierrez J. Periodontal therapy may reduce the risk of preterm low birth weight in women with periodontal disease: a randomized controlled trial. J Periodontol 2002;73:911–24.

ELSEVIER
SAUNDERS

Obstet Gynecol Clin N Am
32 (2005) 411–428

OBSTETRICS AND
GYNECOLOGY
CLINICS
OF NORTH AMERICA

Preterm Premature Rupture of the Membranes: Current Approaches to Evaluation and Management

Brian M. Mercer, MD

Department of Reproductive Biology, Case Western Reserve University, MetroHealth Medical Center,
Suite G240, 2500 MetroHealth Drive, Cleveland, OH 44109, USA

Preterm premature rupture of the membranes (PROM) complicates 3% of pregnancies and is responsible for approximately one third of all preterm births [1–4]. As a result, approximately 150,000 women suffer this pregnancy complication annually in the United States. Preterm PROM is associated with brief latency from membrane rupture to delivery. Particularly when PROM occurs remote from term, there are significant risks of infant morbidity and mortality after birth. Because of the association between PROM and intrauterine infection, oligohydramnios, and placental abruption, the fetus is also at risk before delivery, particularly if conservative management is attempted to prolong the pregnancy.

Because preterm PROM presents a clinical situation where early delivery is to be anticipated and prenatal and neonatal complications are common, the physician caring for women with this common obstetric disorder has an opportunity to intervene in a manner that can improve perinatal outcome. This article addresses clinically relevant questions regarding the evaluation and management of preterm PROM.

Why does preterm premature rupture of the membranes occur?

At term, membrane rupture is a normal part of parturition and can occur before or after the onset of contractions. This results from a combination of cellular apoptosis (programmed cell death), increased collagenase activity, and dissolution of the amniochorionic extracellular matrix, all of which can be exacerbated

---

Reprints are not available.

0889-8545/05/$ – see front matter © 2005 Elsevier Inc. All rights reserved.
doi:10.1016/j.ogc.2005.03.003

by contraction-induced shearing forces [5,6]. In many cases of preterm PROM, it is likely that the same physiologic processes are in place.

With decreasing gestational age of preterm PROM, however, it is more likely that membrane rupture is associated with an underlying pathologic process. Intrauterine infection, as demonstrated by positive amniotic fluid cultures and histologic chorioamnionitis, is common with preterm PROM, particularly with membrane PROM remote from term. It has been suggested that intrauterine infection results from ascending genital tract colonization, leading to increased cytokine activity that enhances membrane apoptosis, production of proteases, and dissolution of the membrane's extracellular matrix [7–9]. Mechanical stretch, as is seen with multiple gestations and polyhydramnios, may enhance local expression of cytokines to increase protease production and could also cause shearing strain on the membranes. Placental abruption could increase decidual-chorionic protease production and dissolution of the extracellular matrix through decidual thrombin expression. Clinical factors associated with PROM include low socioeconomic status and low maternal body mass index, prior preterm birth or preterm labor in the current pregnancy, maternal smoking, urinary tract and sexually transmitted infections, cervical conization or cerclage, and amniocentesis [1–10]. Ultimately, in many cases of preterm PROM, the actual cause of membrane weakening and rupture is not known. It is probable that a number of factors and a maternal genetic or physiologic predisposition act together to cause preterm PROM in many cases.

What is the typical clinical course after preterm premature rupture of the membranes?

Latency from membrane rupture to delivery is generally brief and is inversely proportional to gestational age at membrane rupture. Of all patients with ruptured membranes before 34 weeks of gestation, 93% deliver in less than 1 week [11]. Even with conservative management, at least one half of women deliver within a week of membrane rupture. When women with preterm PROM remote from term are given antibiotics during conservative management (see later), about one half of those remaining pregnant deliver in each subsequent week. Alternatively, a minority of women can benefit from extended latency with conservative management and a small proportion of women with membrane rupture can anticipate cessation of fluid leakage (2.6%–13%), particularly if PROM occurs as a complication of amniocentesis [12,13].

What are the maternal risks associated with preterm premature rupture of the membranes?

Women with preterm PROM and prolonged membrane rupture are at increased risk for chorioamnionitis, which may result from ascending bacterial colonization before membrane rupture (causing PROM) or after membrane rupture (complicating PROM). The risk of infection increases with decreasing gestational age at membrane rupture [14,15], and with increasing duration of membrane rupture. In one study, 9% of women with PROM at term developed chorioamnionitis [16], and the risk increased to 24% with membrane rupture more than 24 hours. With PROM remote from term, chorioamnionitis is common (13%–60%), and postpartum endometritis complicates 2% to 13% of these pregnancies [17,18]. The incidence of placental abruption varies between studies (4%–12%) [19–21]. This is a significantly higher risk than the background population risk (approximately 1 in 200 pregnancies). Serious complications of PROM that have been reported with conservative management of PROM occurring early in pregnancy are retained placenta or postpartum hemorrhage necessitating dilation and curettage (12%); maternal sepsis (0.8%); and death (0.14%) [21].

What are the fetal and neonatal risks of preterm premature rupture of the membranes?

Fetal morbidity after preterm PROM results from maternal intrauterine infection, umbilical cord compression, placental abruption, and prolonged fetal compression caused by oligohydramnios. Each of these places the fetus at increased risk for fetal death (generally approximately 1% with conservative management after the limit of potential neonatal viability) and perinatal asphyxia. The pregnancy complicated by PROM before the limit of fetal viability (currently <23 weeks) is at increased risk for fetal demise (15%); however, a portion of this increase is attributable to nonintervention for fetal benefit when delivery occurs before there is any hope of postnatal survival. When membrane rupture occurs well before the limit of fetal viability (particularly when there is persistent oligohydramnios), there is a significant risk of lethal fetal pulmonary hypoplasia caused by arrested alveolar development. This becomes evident with failure of lung growth despite prolonged latency (see later). Prolonged compression can lead to fetal restriction deformities, similar to those seen in Potter's syndrome. There is accumulating evidence that in utero exposure to infection increases the risk of long-term neurologic sequelae [15], although there are not current data to demonstrate that delivery before the onset of clinical symptoms of infection prevents these adverse outcomes.

The primary determinant of infant morbidity and mortality is gestational age at delivery. In general, infant morbidity can be anticipated to be similar to that of other infants born at the same gestational age (absent pulmonary hypoplasia). Umbilical cord compression before and during labor and placental abruption, however, theoretically increase this risk of hypoxic insult. Additionally, the risk of neonatal infection is approximately twofold higher at any gestational age when delivery occurs after preterm PROM than for other causes. Group B streptococcus is a significant cause of early onset neonatal sepsis and is more likely to occur in the setting of premature birth, prolonged membrane rupture, or amnionitis, each of which is seen commonly with preterm PROM. Lethal pulmonary hypoplasia is rare with PROM, occurring after 24 to 26 weeks' gestation, presumably because alveolar development by this time is adequate to support postnatal life. With PROM remote from term, however, there is the potential for nonlethal pulmonary hypoplasia, manifesting through postnatal pulmonary complications including pneumothorax, pneumomediastinum, and the need for high ventilatory pressures to compensate for poor pulmonary compliance.

In general survival is likely and long-term sequelae uncommon with delivery at or after 32 weeks' gestation (unless PROM occurs before 24–26 weeks' gestation). This is not a distinct cutoff, but rather a continuum with some infants doing well despite earlier delivery and a small number of infants having poor outcomes with delivery near term.

What are the most important determinants of management after preterm premature rupture of the membranes?

Under certain circumstances, delivery is indicated after preterm PROM, regardless of gestational age. Those with advanced labor, evident chorioamnionitis, nonreassuring fetal testing, overt fetal distress or demise, or significant bleeding from placental abruption require expeditious delivery, either vaginally or by cesarean section, as clinically appropriate. When there is significant cervical dilatation and fetal malpresentation, the risk of umbilical cord prolapse increases and may warrant delivery because of the increased risk of fetal loss despite early gestational age.

If the mother and fetus are clinically stable after initial assessment, gestational age is of primary importance in determining management. With preterm PROM, there is potential advantage to conservative management to prolong the latency from membrane rupture to delivery. The immature fetus can benefit if conservative measures prolong the pregnancy adequately to reduce gestational age–dependent morbidity. Alternatively, even brief pregnancy prolongation can benefit the immature fetus if active measures to enhance fetal maturation are undertaken (eg, maternal steroid administration). Once the fetus is mature, there is little to be gained from conservative management after membrane rupture.

What evaluations should be considered for women with preterm premature rupture of the membranes?

The first step in patient evaluation is confirmation of the diagnosis. In most cases, the diagnosis can be made based on history and physical examination. In the setting of a suspicious clinical history, the presence of Nitrazine-positive fluid (pH > 6) passing from the cervix is diagnostic. If the sterile speculum examination is equivocal, a specimen can be collected from the posterior fornix of the vagina with a sterile swab. The swab is then applied to a microscope slide for visualization of "arborized" crystals under low-power microscopy after drying. False-positive results on Nitrazine testing can occur with blood or semen contamination, alkaline antiseptics, or bacterial vaginosis. The ferning test may be falsely positive if there is contamination with cervical mucous (generally nonbranching arborization). False-negative visual examination, ferning, or Nitrazine testing can occur with prolonged leakage with minimal residual fluid. If clinical suspicion remains after initial assessment, the patient can be retested after prolonged recumbency or alternate measures can be considered. A variety of ancillary techniques for confirmation of membrane rupture have been suggested (eg, cervicovaginal fetal fibronectin, human chorionic gonadotropin, maternal serum alpha fetoprotein, among others). These are nonspecific reflecting decidual disruption rather than membrane rupture. A negative test is likely reassuring, but a positive test does not confirm membrane rupture with certainty. Ultrasound evaluation should be performed if the diagnosis is suspected but cannot be confirmed clinically. Oligohydramnios without evident fetal urinary tract malformations or fetal growth restriction may be suggestive of membrane rupture, but is not diagnostic. The diagnosis can be made unequivocally with ultrasound-guided amnioinfusion of indigo carmine (1 mL in 9 mL of sterile normal saline). The passage of blue fluid per vagina onto a perineal pad is confirmatory.

Gestational age should be established based on clinical history and ultrasound. Ultrasound should estimate gestational age if no prior ultrasound has been performed. Even if prior ultrasound has been performed, ultrasound should be considered to assess fetal growth; position; residual amniotic fluid volume; and to identify gross fetal abnormalities, which may cause PROM by hydramnios. The patient should also be evaluated for evidence of advanced labor, chorioamnionitis, placental abruption, or fetal distress. Women with these complications require expeditious delivery.

At the time of initial speculum examination the cervix should be inspected visually for evident cervicitis or umbilical cord or fetal extremity prolapse. Cervical dilatation and effacement can be evaluated visually (correlation coefficient with digital examination, 0.74). To reduce the risk of infectious morbidity, digital examinations should be avoided unless delivery is expected [22]. Cervical cultures (eg, endocervical *Chlamydia trachomatis* and *Neisseria gonorrhoeae*) are appropriate if not previously obtained. Anovaginal cultures for group B streptococcus (*Streptococcus agalactiae*) should be obtained if these have not been performed within the prior 6 weeks.

Where should conservative management be undertaken?

Unless delivery is immediately required, the patient with preterm PROM is best served by care in a facility capable of providing emergent delivery for maternal complications, such as placental abruption, fetal malpresentation in labor, or fetal distress caused by umbilical cord compression or in utero infection.

The facility should also be capable of providing emergent neonatal resuscitation and intensive care. If the initial facility lacks these capabilities, and delivery is not imminent, the patient should be transferred before additional complications occur.

How should the patient with preterm premature rupture of the membranes near term (32–36 weeks) be managed?

The potential for severe acute neonatal morbidity and mortality is low when delivery occurs at 34 to 36 weeks' gestation [23]. Corticosteroids are generally not given to accelerate fetal pulmonary maturity after 34 weeks. Conservative management of PROM at 34 to 36 weeks increases the risks of chorioamnionitis (16% versus 2%, $P = .001$) and lower umbilical cord blood pH (7.35 versus 7.25, $P = .009$), and increases maternal hospital stay (5.2 versus 2.6 days, $P = .006$). Such management has not been shown to significantly reduce neonatal morbidity [24]. Women with PROM at 34 to 36 weeks' gestation should be delivered expeditiously. It is appropriate to transfer these women, before delivery, to a facility capable of caring for an infant delivered at this gestation.

At 32 to 33 weeks' gestation, neonatal survival with immediate delivery is likely. There remains a risk, however, of respiratory distress syndrome (RDS) and other gestational age–dependent morbidities should fetal pulmonary maturity testing be immature. If fetal maturity testing is positive, however, the likelihood of pulmonary and other acute major morbidities is low. In a study of PROM at 32 to 36 weeks' gestation, Mercer et al [25] found no cases of RDS, intraventricular hemorrhage, or necrotizing enterocolitis occurred with documented fetal pulmonary maturity at 32 to 36 weeks' gestation. Alternatively, in that population conservative management prolonged pregnancy only briefly (36 versus 14 hours, $P < .001$); increased the risk of chorioamnionitis (27.7% versus 10.9%, $P = .06$); and increased the risk for occult cord compression, without reducing neonatal morbidity [25]. Similar patterns were seen for those with PROM at 32 to 33 weeks' gestation. In a similar study among a higher-risk population at 30 to 33 weeks' gestation, Cox et al [26] found conservative management prolonged latency only briefly (59% versus 100% delivered at 48 hours, $P < .001$), and increased the risk of chorioamnionitis sevenfold (15% versus 2%, $P = .009$) with no evident reduction in gestational age–dependent morbidity, when tocolysis, antibiotics, and antenatal corticosteroids were not given [26]. In addition, there was one stillbirth caused by suspected occult umbilical cord compression.

When PROM occurs at 32 to 33 weeks' gestation, fetal pulmonary maturity testing should be attempted, if feasible. This can be obtained from vaginal pool or amniocentesis specimens if residual fluid permits. Phosphatidyl glycerol, fetal lung maturity-testing, and lecithin-sphingomyelin ratios are appropriate in this setting. Blood and meconium may lead to falsely immature results, so a mature result is reassuring. Alternatively, if there is significant blood or meconium present, serious consideration should be given to delivery rather than conservative management. If fetal pulmonary maturity is documented, it is generally best to proceed to delivery before infectious complications ensue. If fetal pulmonary immaturity is suspected at 32 to 33 weeks, or should fluid for testing be unavailable, conservative management with close fetal monitoring, adjunctive antibiotic therapy, and antenatal corticosteroid administration (see later) is appropriate. If there is no plan either to induce fetal maturation with corticosteroids or to prolong pregnancy and suppress infection with concurrent antibiotics, however, these patients may be better delivered expeditiously before additional complications occur because extended latency is not likely.

What should be done after corticosteroid benefit has been achieved with antenatal corticosteroids at 32 to 33 weeks gestation?

Once corticosteroid benefit has been achieved after 48 hours of conservative management (see later), the remaining potential for fetal-neonatal benefit is limited unless extended latency of 1 week or more is anticipated. Data regarding the optimal time to discontinue conservative management of PROM are limited. Many physicians proceed to delivery at 34 weeks' gestation. In this scenario, women achieving the benefit of antenatal corticosteroids greater than 33 weeks and 0 days do not accrue benefits of extended latency with delivery a few days later at 34 weeks' gestation, but do incur the risks of chorioamnionitis, umbilical cord compression, and placental abruption. These women are likely best served by delivery once corticosteroid benefit has been achieved. Alternatively, for women with PROM before 33 weeks, or who are cared for at an institution that attempts to prolong latency further than 34 weeks, ongoing conservative management may be appropriate. An alternative approach to management of the woman with PROM at 32 to 33 weeks' gestation is to deliver 24–48 hours after antenatal corticosteroid administration to maximize the benefits of corticosteroid administration and avert the risk of subsequent complications.

How should the patient with premature rupture of the membranes remote from term (before 32 weeks' gestation) be managed?

Delivery before 32 weeks' gestation is associated with a significant risk of severe neonatal morbidities and death. In the absence of indications for delivery, women with preterm PROM at 23 to 31 weeks should be managed conservatively to prolong pregnancy and reduce the risk of gestational age–dependent morbidity. Examples of exceptions to this approach are fetal malpresentation, such as transverse lie-back up with coexisting advanced cervical dilatation; maternal HIV; and primary maternal herpes simplex virus infections. These circumstances increase the risks of fetal death caused by cord prolapse and compression, and maternal-fetal transmission, respectively.

After initial assessment, a period of prolonged fetal heart rate and maternal contraction monitoring is recommended to identify umbilical cord compression or nonplacental contractions. These patients should be admitted to a facility capable of providing emergent delivery for placental abruption, fetal malpresentation in labor, or fetal distress caused by umbilical cord compression or in utero infection. If testing is reassuring, and the patient does not require transfer to another facility, the patient can be monitored on an inpatient antepartum ward. Bed rest in pregnancy may increase the risk of deep venous thrombosis. Leg exercises, antiembolic stockings, or prophylactic doses of subcutaneous heparin may be helpful for those on prolonged bed rest [27]. Digital pelvic examinations increase the risk of amnionitis and decrease latency, and should be avoided unless progressive labor is demonstrated or delivery is indicated. Fetal heart rate and uterine contraction monitoring should be performed at least daily because of the risk of umbilical cord compression and fetal demise [28]. Biophysical profile testing may be confounded by oligohydramnios but can be helpful should the nonstress test be equivocal. If testing reveals intermittent mild umbilical cord compression but otherwise reassuring fetal testing, continuous fetal heart rate monitoring should be considered if the patient is not to be delivered. The clinical findings should be reassessed 24 to 48 hours after antenatal corticosteroid administration and delivery considered if intermittent cord compression persists or other nonreassuring findings are evident. Oligohydramnios (low initial amniotic fluid index or maximum vertical amniotic fluid pocket <2 cm) has been associated with brief latency and with increased risk of amnionitis. Amniotic fluid volume does not accurately predict pregnancy outcome, however, and should not be used in deciding whether to attempt conservative management.

Findings suggestive of intrauterine infection should lead to consideration of delivery. Typical findings include the combination of fever greater than or equal to 100.4°F, uterine tenderness, or maternal or fetal tachycardia in the absence of another source of infection. An elevated maternal white blood cell count is supportive of suspicious clinical findings, but may be artificially elevated by recent antenatal corticosteroid administration (within 5–7 days). In general, routine maternal white blood cell counting is not needed. After initial evaluation on admission, follow-up testing can be considered if clinical findings are suspicious but equivocal. Additional supportive information can be obtained through amniocentesis. Amniotic fluid glucose concentration below 16 to 20 mg/dL, a positive Gram stain, or a positive amniotic fluid culture is also suggestive of intra-amniotic infection [29–31].

Can the patient with preterm premature rupture of the membranes be managed as an outpatient?

Hospitalization is generally indicated during conservative management of preterm PROM. Hospitalization encourages bed rest and pelvic rest, and allows frequent evaluation of maternal and fetal condition. In most cases, latency is relatively brief. For those with prolonged latency, however, there remains an increased risk of umbilical cord compression, fetal demise, and intrauterine infection. It has been suggested that health care costs could be reduced through discharge of the stable gravida [32]. The study was small, however, and lacked the power needed adequately to evaluate fetal, infant, and maternal morbidities. In the absence of data confirming a lack of risk with outpatient management after the limit of potential viability, this practice is discouraged. Further study regarding the risks and benefits of home care after preterm PROM is warranted.

When PROM occurs before the limit of potential viability, outpatient management may be appropriate provided the patient has access to hospital and is compliant to pelvic and modified bed rest. Initial inpatient observation may increase the opportunity for membrane resealing, and allows early identification of infection, fetal demise, or abruption. Generally, if discharged after initial observation, these patients are readmitted at the limit of viability for closer monitoring of maternal and fetal status.

How does pulmonary hypoplasia occur and how is it diagnosed?

PROM occurring before the limit of viability, particularly that occurring before 20 weeks' gestation, is associated with a significant risk of fetal pulmonary hypoplasia. A number of theories have been proposed regarding the mechanism of pulmonary hypoplasia. It is probable, however, that intrauterine pressure supports the tracheobronchial tree, and that either local pulmonary or amniotic fluid factors support alveolar development. Membrane rupture leads to pulmonary collapse with subsequent arrest in alveolar development. This model is supported by animal studies in which amniorrhexis resulted in fetal pulmonary hypoplasia, but amniorrhexis with concurrent tracheal clipping did not.

The process of pulmonary hypoplasia is one that takes time to become apparent subsequent to the initial insult. Over a period of weeks, the lungs fail to grow in pace with the remainder of the fetus. This is manifest on ultrasound as a lag in chest circumference, chest-abdomen ratio, or lung length, among other indirect parameters of pulmonary growth [15,33,34]. Because the lag in lung growth likely reflects the results of an earlier insult rather than an ongoing process, it is unlikely that earlier delivery enhances outcome once pulmonary hypoplasia is suspected.

A variety of treatments to seal the membrane leak (eg, amnioinfusion, and fibrin-platelet-cryoprecipitate or gel-foam sealing) after PROM before viability have been attempted [35–37]. The efficacy and risks of these approaches have not been adequately evaluated to suggest their incorporation into clinical practice.

What are the considerations regarding group B streptococcus prophylaxis after premature rupture of the membranes?

The benefits of intrapartum prophylaxis with intravenous penicillin to prevent maternal-fetal transmission of group B streptococcus (*S agalactiae*) have been well demonstrated [38]. Preterm birth and prolonged membrane rupture are both risk factors for neonatal group B streptococcus sepsis. The patient with preterm PROM should receive intrapartum group B streptococcus prophylaxis unless there is an available recent negative anovaginal culture. Known group B streptococcus carriers should receive intrapartum group B streptococcus prophylaxis regardless of prior treatment. Treatment consists of intravenous penicillin as a 5 million unit initial bolus followed by 2.5 million units every 4 hours, or ampicillin, 2 g then 1 g every 4 hours. Women who are penicillin allergic should be treated with intravenous cefazolin (2 g then 1 g every 8 hours) unless the patient is at significant risk for anaphylaxis or complications should anaphylaxis occur. Under that circumstance, either 500 mg intravenous erythromycin every 6 hours or 900 mg intravenous clindamycin every 8 hours should be given if sensitivity has been demonstrated. In the presence of significant anaphylaxis risk with penicillin and evident resistance to erythromycin or clindamycin, 1 g vancomycin should be given intravenously every 12 hours. The patient who has had a negative anovaginal culture within 6 weeks does not require intrapartum antibiotics unless there is evidence of chorioamnionitis or another medical condition requiring treatment.

Should antibiotics be given to prolong pregnancy and reduce infant morbidity?

This is perhaps one of the best studied areas regarding the treatment of preterm PROM. Over two dozen studies have been published regarding this issue, and most of these have been prospective randomized trials. The goal of adjunctive antibiotic therapy during conservative management of preterm PROM remote from term is to treat or prevent ascending decidual infection to prolong pregnancy and prevent amnionitis and reduce the risk of neonatal sepsis. These studies have been reviewed in a number of meta-analyses and recent publications [12,39,40]. In summary, broad-spectrum antibiotic treatment of conservatively managed women with PROM remote from term prolongs pregnancy, reducing the risk of delivery at 1, 2, and 3 weeks by half. Further, such treatment has been shown to reduce maternal chorioamnionitis, neonatal sepsis, and intraventricular hemorrhage, in addition to reducing the need for neonatal oxygen and surfactant therapy [40].

What is the optimal antibiotic regimen during conservative management of premature rupture of the membranes remote from term?

A number of different antibiotic regimens have been considered in trials addressing this issue. Ultimately, the goal is to provide antibiotic coverage against a range of gram-positive and gram-negative organisms that have been demonstrated in intra-amniotic infections after PROM [21]. At the same time, there is a desire to limit the duration of therapy in the belief that this reduces selection of resistant organisms. Two large multicenter trials highlight different approaches to this issue [41,42]. The National Institutes of Child Health and Human Development Maternal Fetal Medicine Research Units (NICHD-MFMU) Network study of PROM from 24 to 32 weeks' gestation used initial aggressive intravenous therapy (48 hours) with ampicillin (2 g intravenously every 6 hours) and erythromycin (250 mg intravenously every 6 hours), followed by limited duration oral therapy (5 days) with amoxicillin (250 mg orally every 8 hours) and enteric coated erythromycin-base (333 mg orally every 8 hours). These agents provide broad-spectrum antimicrobial coverage and have demonstrated safety when used in pregnancy. Group B streptococcus carriers were treated with ampicillin for 1 week and then again in labor [41,43]. Another multicenter study (The ORACLE trial) included four study arms assigned to oral erythromycin, amoxicillin-clavulanic acid, both, or placebo for up to 10 days after preterm PROM occurring before 37 weeks [42].

The NICHD-MFMU study of PROM from 24 to 32 weeks found that antibiotic treatment increased twofold the likelihood that women would remain undelivered after 7 days of treatment, and that this effect persisted for up to 3 weeks after discontinuation of antibiotics at day 7 [41,43]. These data confirm that antibiotics improved neonatal outcomes including reductions in composite morbidity (one or more of death, RDS, early sepsis, severe intraventricular hemorrhage, or severe necrotizing enterocolitis: 44% versus 53%, $P<.05$), and also individual morbidities, such as RDS (40.5% versus 48.7%), severe necrotizing enterocolitis (2.3% versus 5.8%), patent ductus arteriosus (11.7% versus 20.2%), and chronic lung disease (bronchopulmonary dysplasia: 13% versus 20.5%) ($P \leq .05$ for each). Antibiotic treatment also reduced the incidences of amnionitis (23% versus 32.5%, $P=.01$) and neonatal group B streptococcus sepsis (0% versus 1.5%, $P=.03$). Neonatal sepsis (8.4% versus 15.6%, $P=.009$) and pneumonia (2.9% versus 7%, $P=.04$) were reduced in those who were not group B streptococcus carriers (group B streptococcus carriers received ampicillin even if assigned to placebo).

The ORACLE trial revealed brief pregnancy prolongation (not significant at 7 days), and decreased need for supplemental oxygen (31.1% versus 35.6%, $P=.02$) and positive blood cultures (5.7% versus 8.2%, $P=.02$), but no significant reduction in the primary outcome (composite morbidity: one or more of death, chronic lung disease, or major cerebral abnormality on ultrasonography, 12.7% versus 15.2%, $P=.08$) with erythromycin therapy [42]. Oral amoxicillin–clavulanic acid prolonged pregnancy (43.3% versus 36.7% undelivered after 7 days, $P=.005$) and reduced the need for supplemental oxygen (30.1% versus 35.6%, $P=.05$), but was associated with an increased risk of necrotizing enterocolitis (1.9% versus 0.5%, $P=.001$) without reducing other neonatal complications. The combination of oral amoxicillin–clavulanic acid and erythromycin yielded similar findings. Although oral erythromycin was effective in reducing infant complications, many need to be treated with oral erythromycin to prevent one adverse outcome, given the relatively small differences in outcomes between groups.

The ORACLE trial has raised concern that amoxicillin–clavulanic acid might increase the risk of neonatal necrotizing enterocolitis. This finding is somewhat at odds with the NICHD-MFMU trial, which found a reduction in stage 2 to 3 necrotizing enterocolitis with aggressive antibiotic therapy in a higher-risk population. Overall, the most recent meta-analysis did not find an increased risk of necrotizing enterocolitis with antibiotics, but it is prudent to avoid amoxicillin–clavulanic acid, and also to reduce exposure to any broad-spectrum antibiotics (and chorioamnionitis) by delivering women with PROM near term expeditiously.

It has been questioned whether the duration of antibiotic therapy might be decreased to reduce the potential selection of resistant microorganisms [44,45]. The two prospective studies that have addressed this did not demonstrate increased neonatal risk with shorter duration therapy, and also did not demonstrate less effect on latency than more prolonged therapy. Alternatively, neither study had an adequate sample size and power to demonstrate equivalence between the studied regimens. As such, the NICHD-MFMU protocol of 7 days of therapy is currently recommended.

Because of the several possible indications for antibiotic treatment in this population, attention should be given to avoidance of duplicate treatments. Where possible, antibiotic treatment should include the least number of different antibiotics, in adequate dosages for the identified indications. For example, the patient with evident chorioamnionitis who is receiving intravenous ampicillin and gentamicin or the patient being treated with intravenous cephazolin intrapartum for a concurrent urinary tract infection, does not require additional group B streptococcus therapy with penicillin. The patient receiving ampicillin and erythromycin for pregnancy prolongation that is identified to also have C trachomatis should be treated with erythromycin in adequate dosage to be effective for both indications.

How should the patient with preterm premature rupture of the membranes and cerclage be managed?

Cervical cerclage, particularly emergent cerclage, is a common risk factor for PROM [9,46,47]. There are a number of retrospective studies but no prospective trials regarding the optimal management of PROM with a cervical cerclage in place. It has been found that the risk of adverse perinatal outcomes after PROM with a cerclage is similar to that seen when there is no cerclage in place if the stitch is removed on presentation [48,49]. Studies comparing cerclage retention versus removal after preterm PROM have been small [50–52]. Although these studies seem to have conflicting results, there are several consistent patterns. First, each has found insignificant trends toward increased maternal infection with retained cerclage, and one study found increased infant mortality and death from sepsis with retained cerclage, despite brief pregnancy prolongation. Second, no controlled study has found a significant reduction in infant morbidity with cerclage retention after preterm PROM. Given potential risk without evident neonatal benefit, it is recommended that cerclage be removed on presentation with PROM, particularly if the history of cervical incompetence is equivocal. It may be appropriate to leave the stitch in place during antenatal corticosteroid administration, with removal at 24 to 48 hours, but the benefit of this approach has not been confirmed. If cerclage is retained under this circumstance it is prudent to give concurrent broad-spectrum antibiotics as described previously.

Should antenatal corticosteroids be given in the setting of preterm premature rupture of the membranes?

Antenatal corticosteroid administration should be considered concurrent to conservative management of preterm PROM. These patients are considered to be at significant risk for perinatal morbidity (otherwise they should be delivered). Two recent prospective trials of antenatal corticosteroids concurrent to antibiotic administration have found less RDS (18.4% versus 43.6%, $P = .03$) and no evident increase in perinatal infection (3% versus 5%, $P = $ NS) with antenatal corticosteroids after preterm PROM at 24 to 34 weeks [53], and less perinatal death with treatment for those remaining pregnant at least 24 hours after initiation of treatment (1.3% versus 8.3%, $P = .05$) without an apparent reduction in RDS [54]. The most recently published meta-analysis in this regard has found antenatal corticosteroids during conservative management of PROM to substantially reduce the risks of RDS (20% versus 35.4%), intraventricular hemorrhage (7.5% versus 15.9%), and necrotizing enterocolitis (0.8% versus 4.6%), without significantly increasing the risks of maternal (9.2% versus 5.1%) or neonatal (7% versus 6.6%) infection [55]. Antenatal corticosteroids, either a single course of betamethasone (12 mg intramuscularly, every 24 hours × 2 doses) or dexamethasone (6 mg intramuscularly, every 12 hours × 4 doses), should be administered during conservative management if they have not been previously given.

It has been suggested women with PROM would deliver too quickly to benefit from antenatal corticosteroid administration. This is clearly not the case, because most remain pregnant at least 48 hours, regardless of concurrent antibiotic administration. It has also been suggested that preterm PROM itself might accelerate fetal pulmonary maturation. This is controversial, and even if true, RDS remains the most common acute morbidity in this setting (41% in the NICHD-MFMU trial) [41]. Finally, it has been suggested that antenatal corticosteroid treatment might increase the risk of neonatal infection. This has not been confirmed in meta-analyses, and review of individual studies has revealed no consistent pattern toward increased or decreased infection. With antibiotic treatment, most conservatively managed women with preterm PROM remain pregnant for at least 24 to 48 hours and the risk of infection is decreased. It is prudent to give concurrent broad-spectrum antibiotics as noted previously to prolong pregnancy and reduce infectious morbidity in this situation.

Should tocolytic therapy be used after preterm premature rupture of the membranes

Current data do not confirm that tocolytic therapy after preterm PROM reduces infant morbidity and mortality. Because of this, and because of the potential for intrauterine infection in this setting, some caregivers elect not to treat these women with tocolytic agents, and this is appropriate. Alternatively, prophylactic tocolysis after PROM, particularly if contracting (preterm labor) occurred before preterm PROM, has been found briefly to prolong latency. No studies have evaluated tocolysis given concurrently with antenatal corticosteroid and antibiotics administration. It is plausible that short-term pregnancy prolongation with prophylactic tocolysis could enhance the potential for corticosteroid effect and allow time for antibiotics to act against subclinical decidual infection. It is not unreasonable to administer tocolysis under such circumstances. Further study is needed.

Are neurologic complications linked to preterm premature rupture of the membranes?

Increasing evidence has linked intra-amniotic infections to long-term neurologic complications. Cerebral palsy and cystic periventricular leukomalacia have been linked to amnionitis [56]. Elevated amniotic fluid cytokines and fetal systemic inflammation (termed "fetal inflammatory syndrome"), which may accompany maternal-fetal infection, have been associated with periventricular leukomalacia and subsequent cerebral palsy [57–59]. Because early delivery and perinatal infection are commonly seen with PROM, it might be suggested that women with PROM should be delivered regardless of gestational age. It has not been shown, however, that immediate delivery on admission prevents these sequelae. Although there may not be overt infection on presentation with PROM, it is possible that subclinical infection is already present in some cases and that early delivery does not help. Alternatively, for those with PROM remote from term, conservative management with concurrent antibiotic administration does offer the opportunity to reduce gestational age–dependent and infectious complications. Until evidence of the benefits of immediate delivery become available, conservative management with adjunctive antibiotics to reduce the risk of infection is recommended for women with PROM remote from term (<32 weeks). Near term (≥32 weeks), the risk of major acute and chronic morbidity with delivery is low if pulmonary maturity is documented. Antenatal corticosteroids can be given to accelerate fetal maturation if pulmonary testing is unavailable or suggestive of immaturity. Early delivery should be considered for these women, to reduce the risk of exposure to intrauterine infection and subsequent neurologic morbidity.

Summary

When PROM occurs before term, there are a number of interventions to reduce perinatal complications. In general, unless there is an opportunity to reduce gestational age–dependent morbidity or mortality with conservative management through either antenatal corticosteroid administration or extended latency, the patient is best served by expeditious delivery before complications, such as chorioamnionitis, umbilical cord compression, or abruption occur. When conservative management is undertaken, timely antenatal transfer to a center with facilities for maternal observation and neonatal resuscitation or care, in-hospital monitoring to allow monitoring and early intervention for infection, labor, bleeding, and nonreassuring fetal heart rate patterns, antenatal corticosteroid administration to enhance pulmonary maturation and reduce intraventricular hemorrhage, antibiotic treatment to prolong pregnancy and reduce perinatal infections, and intrapartum group B streptococcus prophylaxis in the absence of recent negative anovaginal cultures each offer the opportunity to enhance pregnancy outcomes.

References

[1] Meis PJ, Ernest JM, Moore ML. Causes of low birth weight births in public and private patients. Am J Obstet Gynecol 1987;156:1165–8.

[2] Tucker JM, Goldenberg RL, Davis RO, et al. Etiologies of preterm birth in an indigent population: is prevention a logical expectation? Obstet Gynecol 1991;77:343–7.

[3] Robertson PA, Sniderman SH, Laros Jr RK, et al. Neonatal morbidity according to gestational age and birth weight from five tertiary care centers in the United States, 1983 through 1986. Am J Obstet Gynecol 1992;166:1629–45.

[4] Martin JA, Hamilton BE, Sutton PD, et al. Births: final data for 2002. Natl Vital Stat Rep 2003;52:1–116.

[5] Skinner SJM, Campos GA, Liggins GC. Collagen content of human amniotic membranes: effect of gestation length and premature rupture. Obstet Gynecol 1981;57:487–9.

[6] Lavery JP, Miller CE, Knight RD. The effect of labor on the rheologic response of chorioamniotic membranes. Obstet Gynecol 1982;60:87–92.

[7] Taylor J, Garite T. Premature rupture of the membranes before fetal viability. Obstet Gynecol 1984;64:615–20.

[8] Naeye RL, Peters EC. Causes and consequences of premature rupture of the fetal membranes. Lancet 1980;1:192–4.

[9] Charles D, Edwards WB. Infectious complications of cervical cerclage. Am J Obstet Gynecol 1981;141:1065–70.

[10] Gold RB, Goyert GL, Schwartz DB, et al. Conservative management of second trimester postamniocentesis fluid leakage. Obstet Gynecol 1989;74:745–7.

[11] Mercer B, Arheart K. Antimicrobial therapy in expectant management of preterm premature rupture of the membranes. Lancet 1995;346:1271–9.

[12] Mercer BM. Management of premature rupture of membranes before 26 weeks' gestation. Obstet Gynecol Clin North Am 1992;19:339–51.

[13] Johnson JWC, Egerman RS, Moorhead J. Cases with ruptured membranes that "reseal." Am J Obstet Gynecol 1990;163:1024–32.

[14] Hillier SL, Martius J, Krohn M, et al. A case-control study of chorioamnionic infection and histologic chorioamnionitis in prematurity. N Engl J Med 1988;319:972–8.

[15] Morales WJ. The effect of chorioamnionitis on the developmental outcome of preterm infants at one year. Obstet Gynecol 1987;70:183–6.

[16] Gunn GC, Mishell DR, Morton DG. Premature rupture of the fetal membranes: a review. Am J Obstet Gynecol 1970;106:469–82.

[17] Garite TJ, Freeman RK. Chorioamnionitis in the preterm gestation. Obstet Gynecol 1982;59: 539–45.

[18] Simpson GF, Harbert Jr GM. Use of β-methasone in management of preterm gestation with premature rupture of membranes. Obstet Gynecol 1985;66:168–75.

[19] Gonen R, Hannah ME, Milligan JE. Does prolonged preterm premature rupture of the membranes predispose to abruptio placentae? Obstet Gynecol 1989;74:347–50.

[20] Vintzileos AM, Campbell WA, Nochimson DJ, et al. Preterm premature rupture of the membranes: a risk factor for the development of abruptio placentae. Am J Obstet Gynecol 1987; 156:1235–8.

[21] Mercer BM, Moretti ML, Prevost RR, et al. Erythromycin therapy in preterm premature rupture of the membranes: a prospective, randomized trial of 220 patients. Am J Obstet Gynecol 1992; 166:794–802.

[22] Alexander JM, Mercer BM, Miodovnik M, et al. The impact of digital cervical examination on expectantly managed preterm rupture of membranes. Am J Obstet Gynecol 2000;183:1003–7.

[23] Mercer BM. Preterm premature rupture of the membranes. Obstet Gynecol 2003;101:178–93.

[24] Naef III RW, Allbert JR, Ross EL, et al. Premature rupture of membranes at 34 to 37 weeks' gestation: aggressive versus conservative management. Am J Obstet Gynecol 1998;178:126–30.

[25] Mercer BM, Crocker L, Boe N, et al. Induction versus expectant management in PROM with mature amniotic fluid at 32–36 weeks: a randomized trial. Am J Obstet Gynecol 1993; 82:775–82.

[26] Cox SM, Leveno KJ. Intentional delivery versus expectant management with preterm ruptured membranes at 30–34 weeks' gestation. Obstet Gynecol 1995;86:875–9.

[27] Kovacevich GJ, Gaich SA, Lavin JP, et al. The prevalence of thromboembolic events among women with extended bed rest prescribed as part of the treatment for premature labor or preterm premature rupture of membranes. Am J Obstet Gynecol 2000;182:1089–92.

[28] Moberg LJ, Garite TJ, Freeman RK. Fetal heart rate patterns and fetal distress in patients with preterm premature rupture of membranes. Obstet Gynecol 1984;64:60–4.

[29] Broekhuizen FF, Gilman M, Hamilton PR. Amniocentesis for gram stain and culture in preterm premature rupture of the membranes. Obstet Gynecol 1985;66:316–21.

[30] Romero R, Yoon BH, Mazor M, et al. A comparative study of the diagnostic performance of amniotic fluid glucose, white blood cell count, interleukin-6, and Gram stain in the detection of microbial invasion in patients with preterm premature rupture of membranes. Am J Obstet Gynecol 1993;169:839–51.

[31] Belady PH, Farhouh LJ, Gibbs RS. Intra-amniotic infection and premature rupture of the membranes. Clin Perinatol 1997;24:43–57.

[32] Carlan SJ, O'Brien WF, Parsons MD, et al. Preterm premature rupture of membranes: a randomized study of home versus hospital management. Obstet Gynecol 1993;81:61–4.

[33] Laudy JA, Tibboel D, Robben SG, et al. Prenatal prediction of pulmonary hypoplasia: clinical, biometric, and Doppler velocity correlates. Pediatrics 2002;109:250–8.

[34] Rizzo G, Capponi A, Angelini E, et al. Blood flow velocity waveforms from fetal peripheral pulmonary arteries in pregnancies with preterm premature rupture of the membranes: relationship with pulmonary hypoplasia. Ultrasound Obstet Gynecol 2000;15:98–103.

[35] Sciscione AC, Manley JS, Pollock M, et al. Intracervical fibrin sealants: a potential treatment for early preterm premature rupture of the membranes. Am J Obstet Gynecol 2001;184:368–73.

[36] Quintero RA, Morales WJ, Bornick PW, et al. Surgical treatment of spontaneous rupture of membranes: the amniograft–first experience. Am J Obstet Gynecol 2002;186:155–7.

[37] O'Brien JM, Barton JR, Milligan DA. An aggressive interventional protocol for early mid-trimester premature rupture of the membranes using gelatin sponge for cervical plugging. Am J Obstet Gynecol 2002;187:1143–6.

[38] American College of Obstetricians and Gynecologists. ACOG Committee Opinion: number 279, December 2002. Prevention of early-onset group B streptococcal disease in newborns. Obstet Gynecol 2002;100:1405–12.

[39] Egarter C, Leitich H, Karas H, et al. Antibiotic treatment in premature rupture of membranes and neonatal morbidity: a meta-analysis. Am J Obstet Gynecol 1996;174:589–97.

[40] Kenyon S, Boulvain M, Neilson J. Antibiotics for preterm rupture of the membranes: a systematic review. Obstet Gynecol 2004;104:1051–7.

[41] Mercer B, Miodovnik M, Thurnau G, et al. Antibiotic therapy for reduction of infant morbidity after preterm premature rupture of the membranes: a randomized controlled trial. JAMA 1997; 278:989–95.

[42] Kenyon SL, Taylor DJ, Tarnow-Mordi W, et al. Broad spectrum antibiotics for preterm, prelabor rupture of fetal membranes: the ORACLE I randomized trial. Lancet 2001;357:979–88.

[43] Mercer BM, Goldenberg RL, Das AF, et al. What we have learned regarding antibiotic therapy for the reduction of infant morbidity? Semin Perinatol 2003;27:217–30.

[44] Lewis DF, Adair CD, Robichaux AG, et al. Antibiotic therapy in preterm premature rupture of membranes: are seven days necessary? A preliminary, randomized clinical trial. Am J Obstet Gynecol 2003;188:1413–6 [discussion: 1416–7].

[45] Segel SY, Miles AM, Clothier B, et al. Duration of antibiotic therapy after preterm premature rupture of fetal membranes. Am J Obstet Gynecol 2003;189:799–802.

[46] Treadwell MC, Bronsteen RA, Bottoms SF. Prognostic factors and complication rates for cervical cerclage: a review of 482 cases. Am J Obstet Gynecol 1991;165:555–8.

[47] Harger JH. Comparison of success and morbidity in cervical cerclage procedures. Obstet Gynecol 1990;56:543–8.

[48] Blickstein I, Katz Z, Lancet M, et al. The outcome of pregnancies complicated by preterm rupture of the membranes with and without cerclage. Int J Gynaecol Obstet 1989;28: 237–42.

[49] Yeast JD, Garite TR. The role of cervical cerclage in the management of preterm premature rupture of the membranes. Am J Obstet Gynecol 1988;158:106–10.

[50] Ludmir J, Bader T, Chen L, et al. Poor perinatal outcome associated with retained cerclage in patients with premature rupture of membranes. Obstet Gynecol 1994;84:823–6.

[51] Jenkins TM, Berghella V, Shlossman PA, et al. Timing of cerclage removal after preterm premature rupture of membranes: maternal and neonatal outcomes. Am J Obstet Gynecol 2000; 183:847–52.

[52] McElrath TF, Norwitz ER, Lieberman ES, et al. Perinatal outcome after preterm premature rupture of membranes with in situ cervical cerclage. Am J Obstet Gynecol 2002;187:1147–52.

[53] Lewis DF, Brody K, Edwards MS, et al. Preterm premature ruptured membranes: a randomized trial of steroids after treatment with antibiotics. Obstet Gynecol 1996;88:801–5.

[54] Pattinson RC, Makin JD, Funk M, et al. The use of dexamethasone in women with preterm premature rupture of membranes: a multicentre, double-blind, placebo-controlled, randomised trial. Dexiprom Study Group. S Afr Med J 1999;89:865–70.

[55] Harding JE, Pang J, Knight DB, et al. Do antenatal corticosteroids help in the setting of preterm rupture of membranes? Am J Obstet Gynecol 2001;184:131–9.

[56] Wu YW, Colford Jr JM. Chorioamnionitis as a risk factor for cerebral palsy: a meta-analysis. JAMA 2000;284:1417–24.

[57] Yoon BH, Jun JK, Romero R, et al. Amniotic fluid inflammatory cytokines (interleukin-6, interleukin 1b, and tumor necrosis factor-α), neonatal brain white matter lesions, and cerebral palsy. Am J Obstet Gynecol 1997;177:19–26.

[58] Yoon BH, Romero R, Kim CJ, et al. High expression of tumor necrosis factor-alpha and interleukin-6 in periventricular leukomalacia. Am J Obstet Gynecol 1997;177:406–11.

[59] Yoon BH, Romero R, Yang SH, et al. Interleukin-6 concentrations in umbilical cord plasma are elevated in neonates with white matter lesions associated with periventricular leukomalacia. Am J Obstet Gynecol 1996;174:1433–40.

ELSEVIER
SAUNDERS

Obstet Gynecol Clin N Am
32 (2005) 429–439

OBSTETRICS AND
GYNECOLOGY
CLINICS
OF NORTH AMERICA

Preterm Labor in Twins and High-Order Multiples

John P. Elliott, MD[a,b,*]

[a]*Phoenix Perinatal Associates, a Division of Obstetrix Medical Group of Phoenix,*
1331 N. 75th Street, 275 Phoenix, AZ 85006, USA
[b]*Division of Maternal-Fetal Medicine, Banner Good Samaritan Medical Center,*
1111 East McDowell Road, Phoenix, AZ 85006, USA

Preterm labor (PTL) in a multiple gestation occurs frequently (twins 50% [1], triplets 76% [2], quadruplets 90% [3]) and is a common reason for preterm delivery (PTD) (twins 34%, triplets 58% [2], quads 26.9% [3]). In a large study of twins delivering preterm (between 33 and 36.9 weeks) [4], 22% of the PTDs were considered nonindicated (discretionary). This fact is rather concerning about the management decisions of obstetricians caring for twin gestations. Of the deliveries that had indications, PTL was the reason for delivery in almost two thirds (65.1%) of patients.

Garite and colleagues [5] demonstrated in a large database of newborns (51,388) that gestational age-specific mortality and survival without significant morbidity are similar for singletons, twins, and triplets, establishing that the determining factor affecting neonatal outcome is prematurity. Management strategies for multiple gestations must be directed at early detection of PTL and effective strategies to delay or prevent PTD. Unlike singleton gestation where identification of patients at risk for PTL is often difficult, every multiple gestation is at risk for PTL, so all patients can be managed as being at risk. Although PTL is a significant cause of PTD, one must recognize that there are other reasons for delivery in multiple gestations. Clinicians must treat the whole patient and extend the pregnancy to the most advanced gestational age possible that is consistent with the best outcome. If nutritional needs are not addressed, the incidence of intrauterine growth restriction increases and premature delivery may be indicated

---

* Division of Maternal-Fetal Medicine, Banner Good Samaritan Medical Center, 1111 East McDowell Road, Phoenix, AZ 85006.

E-mail address: John_elliott@obstetrix.com

0889-8545/05/$ – see front matter © 2005 Elsevier Inc. All rights reserved.
doi:10.1016/j.ogc.2005.04.003
obgyn.theclinics.com

for that reason. Similarly, issues with anemia, preeclampsia, diabetes mellitus, and cervical insufficiency may influence the timing of delivery. Although these factors are not the main topic of this article, they do form the context in which PTL occurs [6]. There are three important areas regarding PTL in a multiple gestation that warrant consideration: (1) prevention strategies, (2) early detection of PTL, and (3) treatment of PTL when it occurs. There is an old adage that an ounce of prevention is worth a pound of cure, which is extremely important in managing PTL of multiple gestations. Clinical and research efforts to prevent PTD have generally taken an approach that started at the end of the process when the patient is experiencing PTL. Tocolytic drugs have been used to treat acute PTL, including magnesium sulfate ($MgSO_4$), β-sympathomimetic agents (ritodrine and terbutaline), calcium channel antagonists, and prostaglandin synthetase inhibitors (indomethacin), with varying success. The use of these and other medications for maintenance tocolysis (beyond 48 hours) or as a prophylactic strategy (before PTL has started) has found limited success. The variability in success is certainly caused by many factors including multiple etiologies for PTL (infection, uterine distention, placental vascular changes [abruption, thrombophilia], premature rupture of membranes, cervical insufficiency, nutrition, and idiopathic); identification of patients at risk; early diagnosis; choice of drugs for treatment; and aggressiveness in the use of the tocolytic therapy.

Efforts to make the diagnosis of PTL early in the process have been successful using home contraction monitoring (HOM) [7], but the impact on PTD has been limited by ineffective strategies to maintain the pregnancy beyond acute tocolysis. Risk identification by history (eg, prior PTL with PTD, prior premature rupture of membranes with PTD), anatomy (eg, incompetent cervix or uterine anomaly), diagnostic testing (eg, fetal fibronectin), or cervical length measurement has also been limited by lack of effective management strategies. I believe that a better approach to this problem is to focus on the patient who is not in active PTL because that is the end stage of this process. Tocolysis with drugs is the only option then, and there is a significant chance of failure with a PTD resulting. The uterus is a smooth muscle with an innate ability to contract. These contractions occur even when nonpregnant (menstrual contractions). In pregnancy, this inherent uterine contractility is the foundation, which is then acted on by various forces that may cause true PTL. Why do some patients with a given risk factor go into PTL, whereas others do not? With twins, 40% develop PTL and 60% do not. What differentiates Mrs. Smith from Mrs. Jones?

PTL involves contractions and cervical change. If the uterus has the ability to contract, then these contractions can be measured. These contractions can be organized conceptually using a device called a "contraction-stat." This is similar to a thermostat. A thermostat responds to external forces (a finger), which then act on a switch, which affects the central heating-cooling machinery causing the room to become warmer or cooler. Similarly, external forces can act on the uterus to produce a change in the number of contractions. If a patient complains infrequently of syncope, an EKG is unlikely to detect an arrhythmia. An extended period of observation (Holter Monitor) may be more successful in detection of

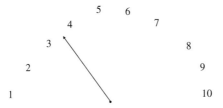

Fig. 1. Illustration of a contraction-stat with 3.5 ctx/h/wk.

the arrhythmia. Monitoring uterine contractions for 2 hours a day does not give as accurate information as 24-hour monitoring, but it seems to be adequate for the need to assess baseline uterine activity. If there is 2 hours of contraction monitoring a day, then each week there is an average of 14 hours of observation and one can determine the contractions (ctx) per hour per week. Repeating that calculation each successive week yields an ongoing assessment of the background contractile activity for that patient. Fig. 1 illustrates a theoretical background average contraction rate of 3.5 ctx/h/wk.

There are many factors that affect the contractility of the uterus (Box 1). Gestational age affects the background contractility. Contractions are visualized

---

Box 1. Factors influencing the contraction-stat

Increasing

Gestational age
Time of day
Estrogen
Uterine stretch
Physical activity
Infection
Placental abruption
Drugs
Stress

Decreasing

Progesterone
Drugs
$MgSO_4$
Betamimetics
Prostaglandin synthetase inhibitors
Calcium channel blocker
Rest
Biofeedback

on ultrasound from conception and increase with gestational age [8,9]. Indeed, these background contractions were described by Braxton-Hicks [10] from the third month until delivery. Frequent contractions (more than five per hour) occurring at less than 36 weeks of gestation are potentially dangerous and should be presumed to be PTL until evaluation proves otherwise. Moore and colleagues [8] showed that uterine activity changes with the time of day. Contractions increase from 5:00 PM to 3:00 AM because of the normal diurnal release of cortisol from the adrenal gland. Endogenous hormones also have an effect on uterine activity. Estrogen increases contractions by increasing gap junctions (estriol surge) and this is opposed by the effect of progesterone, which acts to inhibit contractions [11,12]. Background uterine activity is affected by excessive uterine stretch (multiple gestation, hydramnios). For any gestational age, the greater the number of fetuses the greater the background contractions [13,14]. Uterine activity is increased by physical activity [15] and is decreased by bed rest, although bed rest alone has not been shown to prevent PTL. Infection can cause uterine contractions and PTL in some pregnant women. Cystitis, pyelonephritis, and appendicitis [16] can all affect contractions and there are associations with vaginal infections (bacterial vaginosis). Physical stress (either at work or at home) and psychologic stress can increase contractions. I have used biofeedback techniques to reduce contractions in some patients.

Finally, numerous drugs affect uterine contractions. Some act to increase contractions (eg, oxytocin, prostaglandin preparations, misoprostol, and ergot alkaloids), whereas other drugs inhibit contractions (eg, $MgSO_4$, betamimetics [terbutaline and ritodrine], prostaglandin synthetase inhibitors [indomethacin, ibuprofen, ketorolac tromethamine, and so forth], and calcium channel antagonists [nifedipine]). Some drugs have an indirect stimulatory effect on the uterus. For instance betamethasone, given to enhance pulmonary maturity, increases contractions in triplet and quadruplet pregnancies [17] and can cause PTD.

I propose that the higher the background contraction rate, the greater the risk of PTL developing. Is there a threshold of background uterine activity that is potentially dangerous? Although there are no studies available that have formally addressed this issue, there are several observations that might be informative. Garite et al [13] observed that the mean uterine activity 48 hours before PTL was 3.5 ctx/h, which increased to 5.5 ctx/h 24 hours before the initiation of PTL. Newman and colleagues [18] found a subtle increase in background contractions (0.5 ctx/h/d) before PTL starting 6 days before PTL occurred. The mean contractions 24 hours before PTL were 3.2/h in their study. A separate observation was made by Elliott and Radin [17] in high-order multiple gestations when their data on the effect of betamethasone on contractions was published. Contractions increased after steroid administration with a peak in activity 18 hours after the first dose. If the background uterine activity (before steroids) was less than 3.5 ctx/h, an increase in contractions was observed without cervical change or delivery. In HOM gestations with a background frequency of greater than or equal to 3.5 ctx/h, there was a statistically significant increase in cervical change and in PTD. Based on these observations, I suggest 3.5 ctx/h as a possible threshold value to be used in multifetal gestation.

Returning to the fundamental question of why some patients with multiple gestation (or any other risk factor) develop PTL, whereas others do not, PTL seems to be an episodic event, which starts and if it is successfully treated stops until some event triggers PTL again. If PTL is considered greater than or equal to 8 ctx/h with cervical change, it makes sense that the closer one is to that level of contractions (eg, 5 ctx/h), the greater the chance the patient will go into PTL. Conversely, the quieter the uterus (eg, 1.1 ctx/h) the greater the stimulus that is needed to cause greater than or equal to 8 ctx/h. If the amount of uterine activity associated with various forces acting on the contraction-stat could be determined, a model for PTL could be developed. For example, one could say that bacterial vaginosis is going to cause 2 ctx/h; dehydration 3 ctx/h; shopping at the mall for 3 hours, 3 ctx/h; moving into a new house 4 ctx/h; small placental abruption 5 ctx/h; asymptomatic urinary tract infection 4 ctx/h; bacteremia from infection (pyelonephritis, gingival disease, pneumonia) 6 ctx/h; physical abuse 5 ctx/h; and so forth.

In my own theoretic model I have Mrs. Jones pregnant with twins and her contraction-stat shows 2.2 ctx/h at 28 weeks. Mrs. Smith, also pregnant with twins, has a baseline contraction frequency of 5.4 ctx/h at 28 weeks. They decide to go shopping for "baby" stuff. They are at the mall for 4 hours and Mrs. Jones has a water bottle with her, but Mrs. Smith had not been advised to stay well hydrated. Mrs. Smith begins to feel pressure and backache, which she ignores for 2 hours until she becomes uncomfortable. Mrs. Jones drives Mrs. Smith to the hospital where the monitor shows 12 ctx/h (every 5 minutes) and her cervix is 1 cm 50% effaced. Mrs. Jones asks to be monitored also and she is having 5 ctx/h (every 12 minutes) and her cervix was closed. One is in PTL, the other only increased contractions. Why? Mrs. Jones started with a lower baseline and did experience a stressor (increased physical activity) so contractions increased from 2.2 + 3 = 5 ctx/h. Mrs. Smith had a higher background contraction pattern and then superimposed two stresses (increased physical activity, 3 ctx/hr, and dehydration, 3 ctx/hr, resulting in 5.4 ctx/h + 3 ctx/h + 3 ctx/h = 12 ctx/h). This illustrates a potential mechanism discriminating between patients with the same underlying risk for PTL.

How can the concept of a contraction-stat help clinicians to manage PTL in multiple gestations (or any patient)? The role as caregivers for pregnant women (especially multiple gestations) is to aggressively minimize the risk of developing PTL (this includes recurrent PTL once it has been controlled). A potential management strategy is to minimize the background uterine activity on the contraction-stat. Additionally, one attempts to reduce the occurrence of the known stressors that act on the uterus, especially infectious disease. Background contractions occurring below the threshold (3.5 ctx/h/wk) do not necessarily need manipulation, but if the patient exceeds the threshold ($\geq$3.5 ctx/h/wk), interventions are appropriate to lower the contraction-stat to safer levels. This gives a measurable goal to evaluate the success of the manipulation.

Interventions to lower background contractions

Factors that reduce uterine activity are currently limited. Although bed rest has never been shown to prevent PTL or PTD by itself [19], every woman carrying a multiple gestation can verify that bed rest decreases the frequency of contractions. If one tries to fit decreased physical activity into the model, it can be given a decrease of 1.5 ctx/h. This change does not prevent PTD by itself very often, but it may reduce the background activity enough that when the stress occurs contractions increase, but PTL does not occur. Papiernik et al [20] reported that paid work leave in France, which was part of a program of stress reduction, resulted in a decrease in PTD. Psychologic stress or anxiety can cause contractions, probably mediated by hormonal release (fight or flight mechanism). A routine cervical examination in the office of a HOM gestation that reveals cervical change that needs evaluation in the hospital will frequently cause the patient to be having contractions every 3 minutes when she reaches the hospital. I believe it is the sudden realization that there is trouble, with possible delivery occurring, and that her babies are in danger, which initiates the contractions. The role of stress reduction in reducing contractions has not been studied, but anecdotally I have seen biofeedback techniques reduce contractions. Perhaps this is worth 1 ctx/h.

The next possible intervention to decrease the contraction-stat is hormonal. Progesterone has been shown to decrease the incidence of PTD in some categories of patients at risk [12,21,22]. Of interest, da Fonseca and colleagues [22] monitored each patient in their study (prospectively comparing progesterone with placebo for prevention of PTD in singleton gestations at risk) for 1 h/wk compared with 14 h/wk for the contraction-stat. Table 1 reproduces their data concerning mean contractions at each gestational age from 28 to 34 weeks and Table 2 reproduces a comparison of contractions per hour for the whole pregnancy between progesterone and placebo. Note the progression of increasing background contractions in Table 1 in both groups from 28 to 34 weeks. Proges-

Table 1
Mean contraction frequency for each gestational week between placebo and progesterone groups

Gestational age	Placebo mean ± SD	Progesterone mean ± SD	P value
28	4 ± 3	1 ± 0.6	.00001
29	4 ± 2.1	1 ± 0.9	.00001
30	6.2 ± 3	2.8 ± 2.7	.00001
31	5.1 ± 2.5	3.2 ± 2	.0001
32	6.5 ± 3.1	2.5 ± 2.5	.01
33	7 ± 4.2	2.8 ± 2.4	.0001
34	6.5 ± 3.1	3.5 ± 2	.0001

From da Fonseca EB, Bittar RE, Carvalho MHB, et al. Prophylactic administration of progesterone by vaginal suppository to reduce the incidence of spontaneous preterm birth in women at increased risk: a randomized placebo-controlled double-blind study. Am J Obstet Gynecol 2003;188:419–24; with permission.

Table 2
Frequency of uterine contractions

Contraction	Placebo ($n = 70$)	Progesterone ($n = 72$)	P value
<4	32 (45.7%)	55 (87.4%)	.0001
4–5	12 (71.1%)	3 (4.1%)	.0118
≥6	26 (37.2%)	14) 19.4%)	.0190

From da Fonseca EB, Bittar RE, Carvalho MHB, et al. Prophylactic administration of progesterone by vaginal suppository to reduce the incidence of spontaneous preterm birth in women at increased risk: a randomized placebo-controlled double-blind study. Am J Obstet Gynecol 2003;188:419–24; with permission.

terone therapy powerfully decreased the background uterine activity. Of interest also in Table 1 is that the mean contractions per hour are below the threshold value until 34 weeks when it reaches 3.5 ctx/h. In Table 2, progesterone resulted in 76.4% of the patients having less than 4 ctx/h compared with only 45.7% for the placebo patients. Progesterone seems to be acting to lower the background uterine contractions. The incidence of PTL was reported as similar in both groups, which is not consistent with the theory, unless PTL in the progesterone group occurred in the patients with the higher contractions per hour. Progesterone is not currently indicated in multiple gestations for reduction of PTL, but certainly it theoretically fits the contraction-stat model. There are currently two multicenter prospective randomized controlled trials underway to address the use of prophylactic progesterone in multiple gestation.

The final intervention that can be used to lower the background contractions is tocolytic drugs. Tocolytic drugs can be used in acute PTL, as maintenance therapy following successful acute tocolysis, or prophylactically before the development of PTL in patients at risk. Several studies have examined the use of prophylactic tocolysis in twins with β-sympathomimetic drugs [23–26]. Only one [26] found some benefit with oral terbutaline. These reports, and every study involving tocolysis to prevent PTD, do not include a measurable end point to guide dosing of the drug. Patients in these studies were not assessed to determine if uterine contractions had been decreased to any chosen outcome measure (eg, 3.5 ctx/h). Elliott and colleagues [27] reported the prophylactic use of terbu-taline pump tocolysis in HOM gestations. I monitored the background contrac-tions in triplet and quadruplet pregnancies using the threshold value of 3.5 ctx/h to initiate prophylactic tocolysis to decrease contractions. Of 15 triplets and quadruplet pregnancies that received prophylactic tocolysis with a terbutaline pump, 5 (33%) eventually developed PTL, albeit with a mean delay before onset of PTL of 26.4 days. The mean gestational age at the start of the pump was 24.4 ± 3.9 weeks in triplets and 21.1 ± 1.5 weeks in quadruplets emphasizing how early these pregnancies have significant uterine activity. Using this approach, tocolytic failure was the reason for delivery in 2 (13%) of 15 of triplets and 1 (17%) of 6 of the quadruplet pregnancies, which compares favorably with a 58% incidence of PTD caused by PTL reported in triplets by Malone and colleagues [2]. It is important to note that higher doses of terbutaline (basal infusion rate of 0.066–0.076 mg/h, approximately 16% greater than singleton pregnancies) were needed in HOM gestations because of increased renal clearance of the drug. A prospective trial is needed to determine if prophylactic tocolysis (with a goal of maintaining the contraction-stat below 3.5 ctx/h) reduces PTD caused by PTL in multiple gestations.

Although I believe that prevention of PTL should be the goal of therapy, there are patients who develop PTL. PTL in a multiple gestation is very difficult to control with tocolytic drugs once it has started. The increased renal clearance of drugs in multiple gestations, because of increased blood flow to the kidneys, necessitates increased dosage of tocolytic medications in acute PTL. Elliott and Radin [28] published data showing that higher doses of $MgSO_4$ had to be administered to achieve therapeutic serum levels in HOM gestations compared with singleton pregnancy. It is important to remember that therapeutic serum levels are necessary for the tocolytic drug to be successful. Frequently, too little drug is administered to achieve a therapeutic effect and when contractions do not stop, the drug is declared a failure and discontinued when really the dosage only needed to be increased to treat the patient successfully. A prospective study by Cox and colleagues [29] illustrates the danger of giving too little drug and then declaring that the drug is ineffective at preventing PTD.

In my experience acute tocolysis in multiple gestations frequently requires not only higher dosages but also multiple drugs ($MgSO_4$, terbutaline, and indomethacin). I limit intravenous fluids to reduce the risk of pulmonary edema, but am aggressive with all these drugs. The initial bolus of $MgSO_4$ is 6 g and then 3 g/h infusion. I occasionally increase it to as much as 6 g/h infusion, if necessary, monitoring magnesium levels to maintain a serum level of 8.5 mg/dL in resistant cases. Subcutaneous terbutaline can be used as intermittent injection dosing (0.25 mg) or with continuous infusion of a basal rate and programmed periodic boluses by infusion pump. Indomethacin (100-mg suppositories six to eight times) can be added or alternatively ibuprofen, 600 mg every 6 hours, may be used. After 48 to 72 hours with the contractions spaced out to 3 to 5 per hour, the patient can be converted to a terbutaline pump. Oral maintenance tocolysis is generally ineffective, especially in multiple gestations because of the enhanced renal clearance of the drug. Extended tocolysis with continuous intravenous $MgSO_4$ or terbutaline pump is more effective in maintaining the pregnancy than oral agents, especially when the cervix is dilated greater than or equal to 2 cm or the station is -1 or lower. Both $MgSO_4$ and terbutaline pumps can be used for months with minimal side effects, but the former is used inpatient, whereas the latter may be used in the home. The side effects of $MgSO_4$ include headache, chest pressure, warm flushed feeling, nausea, double vision, and muscle weakness. These all disappear at 72 to 96 hours of therapy. Extended home management on terbutaline pump therapy is appropriate in many circumstances.

There is absolutely no evidence that tocolytic drugs lose their efficacy at 48 hours. Physicians have a tendency to decrease drug therapy too soon when the PTL has not resolved, when one should use the drugs aggressively and appropriately to achieve the desired effect. The most feared complication of toco-lytic therapy is pulmonary edema. Pulmonary edema is not caused by the $MgSO_4$, but is related instead to associated cardiovascular stresses. In unpublished data from my practice, every patient who developed pulmonary edema had one or more of the following cardiovascular stressors: fluid overload, hypertension, infection, multiple gestation, or anemia. If pulmonary edema develops, one should decrease the dose of $MgSO_4$ and treat with oxygen and furosemide for diuresis. The drug does not need to be discontinued. The incidence of pulmonary edema is 3% to 5% in multiple gestations on $MgSO_4$. Complications of terbutaline pump therapy are very rare. Elliott et al [30] documented mild transient side effects (tremors, shortness of breath, or chest discomfort) in 15.5% and serious cardio-vascular complications in 12 (0.1%) of 9359, with 9 of the 12 being pulmonary edema. Tocolytics are safe and effective when used by experienced physicians and nurses.

Summary

PTL occurs frequently in multiple gestations and is the reason for delivery in many twins, triplets, and quadruplet pregnancies. Physicians should take a different approach to these complicated pregnancies because what has been done before has not had any effect on the prematurity rate among such patients in the United States. The goal as obstetric providers should be to assess the background uterine activity and establish the contraction-stat. These background contractions must be therapeutically manipulated (if necessary) to keep them below 3.5 ctx/h/wk. If tocolytic therapy is necessary to achieve this contraction frequency, whatever drug prescribed should be titrated to keep the contractions below 3.5/h/wk. Research is needed with tocolytics that are dosed aggressively to achieve a measurable end point (<3.5 ctx/h/wk). Bed rest and stress reduction probably will not prevent PTL as sole therapies, but are adjunctive care to reduce the contraction-stat. The physician should have the philosophy of never giving up. It is not acceptable to have a PTD of a multiple gestation unless the risks of remaining pregnant exceed the risks in the nursery. Ideally, dichorionic twins should deliver at 37 to 38 weeks, monochorionic-diamniotic twins at 36 to 37 weeks, monochorionic-monoamniotic twins at 32 to 34 weeks, triplets at 35 to 36 weeks, and quadruplets at 34 weeks. Clinicians have to want to prevent a PTD to make that happen.

References

[1] Roberts WE, Morrison JC, Hamer CA, et al. The incidence of preterm labor and specific risk factors. Obstet Gynecol 1990;76:85–95.
[2] Malone FD, Kaufman GE, Chelmow D, et al. Maternal morbidity associated with triplet pregnancy. Am J Perinatol 1998;15:73–7.

[3] Francois K, Sears C, Wilson R, et al. Maternal morbidity and obstetrical complications of quadruplet pregnancy: twelve years experience at a single institution. Am J Obstet Gynecol 2001;184:174.

[4] Elliott JP, Istwan NB, Collins A, et al. Indicated and non-indicated preterm delivery in twin gestations: impact on neonatal outcome and cost. J Perinatol 2004;25:4–7.

[5] Garite TJ, Clark RH, Elliott JP, et al. Twins and triplets: The effect of plurality and growth on neonatal outcome compared with singleton infants. Am J Obstet Gynecol 2004;1991: 700–7.

[6] Elliott JP. Management of high-order multiple gestation. Clin Perinatol 2005;32:387–402.

[7] Mou SM, Sunderji SG, Gall S, et al. Multicenter randomized clinical trial of home uterine activity monitoring for detection of preterm labor. Am J Obstet Gynecol 1991;165: 858–66.

[8] Moore TM, Iams JD, Creasy RK, et al. Diurnal and gestational patterns of uterine activity in normal human pregnancy. Obstet Gynecol 1994;83:517.

[9] Main DM, Grisso JA, Wold J, et al. Extended longitudinal study of uterine activity among low-risk women. Am J Obstet Gynecol 1991;165:1317–22.

[10] Braxton-Hicks J. Trans Obstet Soc London 1871;12:216–31.

[11] McGregor JA, Jackson GM, Lachelin GC, et al. Salivary estriol as a risk assessment fore preterm labor: a prospective trial. Am J Obstet Gynecol 1995;173:1337.

[12] Keirse MJNC, Grant A, King JF. Preterm labor. In: Chalners I, Enkin M, Keirse MJNC, editors. Effective care in pregnancy and childbirth. New York: Oxford University Press; 1989. p. 694–745.

[13] Garite TJ, Bentley DL, Hamer CA, et al. Uterine activity characteristics in multiple gestations. Obstet Gynecol 1990;76:56.

[14] Newman RB, Gill PJ, Campion S, et al. The influence of fetal number on antepartum uterine activity. Obstet Gynecol 1989;73:695.

[15] Spinnewijn WEM, Lotgering FK, Struijk PC, et al. Fetal heart rate and uterine contractility during maternal exercise at term. Am J Obstet Gynecol 1996;174:43.

[16] Mourad J, Elliott JP, Erickson L, et al. Appendicitis in pregnancy; new information that contradicts long held clinical belief. Am J Obstet Gynecol 2000;182:1027–9.

[17] Elliott JP, Radin TG. The effect of corticosteroid administration on uterine activity and preterm labor in high-order multiple gestation. Obstet Gynecol 1995;85:250–4.

[18] Newman RB, Istwan NB, Rhea D, et al. Uterine contraction pattern prior to diagnosis of preterm labor with cervical change. Am J Obstet Gynecol 2002;187:S125.

[19] Goldenberg RL, Cliver SP, Bronstein J, et al. Bed rest in pregnancy. Obstet Gynecol 1994; 84:131–6.

[20] Papiernik E, Bouyer J, Dreyfus J, et al. Prevention of preterm births: a perinatal study in Haguenau, France. Pediatrics 1985;76:154–8.

[21] Meis PJ, Klebanoff M, Thom E, et al. Prevention of recurrent preterm delivery by 17 alpha-hydroxy-progesterone caproate. N Engl J Med 2003;348:2379–85.

[22] da Fonseca EB, Bittar RE, Carvalho MHB, et al. Prophylactic administration of progesterone by vaginal suppository to reduce the incidence of spontaneous preterm birth in women at increased risk: a randomized placebo-controlled double-blind study. Am J Obstet Gynecol 2003; 188:419–24.

[23] O'Connor MC, Murphy H, Dairymple IJ. Double blind trial of ritodrine and placebo in twin pregnancy. Br J Obstet Gynaecol 1979;86:706–9.

[24] Marivate M, DeVilliera KO, Fairbrother P. The effect of prophylactic outpatient administration of fenoterol on the time of onset of spontaneous labor and fetal growth rate in twin pregnancy. Am J Obstet Gynecol 1977;128:707.

[25] Skjaerris J, Aber A. Prevention of prematurity in twin pregnancy by orally administered terbutaline. Acta Obstet Gynecol Scand 1982;108:39.

[26] O'Leary JA. Prophylactic tocolysis of twins. Am J Obstet Gynecol 1986;154:904–5.

[27] Elliott JP, Flynn M, Kaemmerer EL, et al. Terbutaline pump tocolysis in high order multiples. J Reprod Med 1997;42:687–93.

[28] Elliott JP, Radin TG. Serum magnesium levels during magnesium sulfate tocolysis in high order multiple gestations. J Reprod Med 1995;40:450.

[29] Cox SM, Sherman LM, Leveno KJ. Randomized investigation of magnesium sulfate for prevention of preterm birth. Am J Obstet Gynecol 1990;163:767.

[30] Elliott JP, Istwan NB, Rhea D, et al. The occurrence of adverse events in women receiving continuous subcutaneous terbutaline therapy. Am J Obstet Gynecol 2004;191:1277–82.

ELSEVIER
SAUNDERS

Obstet Gynecol Clin N Am
32 (2005) 441–456

OBSTETRICS AND
GYNECOLOGY
CLINICS
OF NORTH AMERICA

Does Cerclage Prevent Preterm Birth?

Orion A. Rust, MD*, William E. Roberts, MD

*Division of Maternal Fetal Medicine, Department of OB/GYN, Lehigh Valley Hospital,
Cedar Crest Boulevard and I-78, Allentown, PA 18105, USA*

Cervical surgery to prevent recurrent pregnancy loss was introduced in 1902 by Herman [1], when he reported on his experience of three patients treated by Emmet trachelorrhaphy. In 1955 Shirodkar [2] and later in 1957 McDonald [3] introduced methods of transvaginal cerclage to treat cervical incompetence. Despite minor modifications, these procedures have remained the mainstay of therapy to prevent recurrent pregnancy loss.

Cervical incompetence has been defined as a physical deficit in the strength of the cervical tissue that is either congenital or acquired [4]. Examples of congenital disorders associated with recurrent pregnancy loss include mullerian anomalies, diethylstilbestrol exposure, and Ehlers-Danlos syndrome. Examples of acquired disorders of the cervical stroma that could potentially result in recurring pregnancy loss include obstetric trauma, such as cervical laceration extending into the lower uterine segment, or gynecologic procedures, such as cervical conization. Cervical incompetence has been traditionally diagnosed by the historic criteria of painless dilation of the cervix; recurrent early preterm delivery (<32 weeks) or second-trimester loss; and progressively earlier delivery with each subsequent pregnancy. In the 1990s, with the advent of transvaginal ultrasound and cervical length measurement, sonographic criteria were developed to diagnose cervical incompetence. This included a short closed cervical length; dilation of the internal os; and prolapse of the membranes into the endocervical canal (funneling or beaking). In addition, exacerbations of these findings with transfundal pressure were also considered a hallmark of this disease [5].

---

* Corresponding author.
E-mail address: P8570@LVH.com (O.A. Rust).

0889-8545/05/$ – see front matter © 2005 Elsevier Inc. All rights reserved.
doi:10.1016/j.ogc.2005.04.001

Classification

Treatment for the diagnosis of cervical incompetence has traditionally used a cerclage procedure. The different types of cerclage can be classified with respect to timing in gestation and anatomic approach (Table 1). Kurup and Goldkrand [6] classified the timing of cerclage as being elective, urgent, or emergent. Elective cerclage is defined as placement in the late first trimester or early second trimester (usually less than 16 weeks gestational age), after viability has been established, and the absence of gross congenital anomalies (eg, anencephaly) has been ensured. This type of cerclage is placed before the development of any signs or symptoms of cervical incompetence. An urgent cerclage is usually placed between 16 and 24 weeks gestational age with most patients being asymptomatic. The diagnosis is made by transvaginal ultrasound with dilation of the internal os, prolapse of the fetal membranes into the endocervical canal, and a short cervical length, or by digital examination with demonstrable cervical dilatation or significant change in effacement when compared with first-trimester examination. Emergent cerclage is usually associated with symptoms, such as pelvic pressure or change in vaginal discharge, with fetal membranes prolapsed beyond the external os. The timing is usually between 16 and 24 weeks and this usually represents imminent pregnancy loss unless this process can be stabilized.

The anatomic approaches to cerclage placement can be from the transvaginal or transabdominal route, with transvaginal being the most common approach. Transvaginal cerclage can be further subdivided into a McDonald type or Shirodkar type. The McDonald type of cerclage is a purse-string stitch placed in the stroma of the ectocervix at the level of the cervical reflection of the vaginal fornices. This type of cerclage is the most common type used in the United States today [7]. The McDonald type of cerclage is easily taught and can be used in most circumstances where the cervical anatomy is easily identified. The Shirodkar transvaginal cerclage requires more experience because of the dissection that is involved. An incision of the vaginal mucosa in the anterior and posterior plane is made. The pubocervical fascia at the level of the internal os is identified using sharp or blunt dissection. The purse string stitch is placed into the cervical stroma with the vasculature of the cardinal ligament lateral to the suture on each side. This type of cerclage is preferred for those patients with altered or absent ectocervical anatomy. Various suture materials and anchoring techniques have been advocated for cerclage procedures. At this time, synthetic permanent mono-filament suture or braided permanent tape have been utilized most often. A recent

Table 1
Classification of cerclage procedures

Timing	Anatomic approach
Elective	Transvaginal
Urgent	McDonald type
Emergent	Shirodkar type
	Transabdominal

study demonstrated that the choice of suture had little impact, if any, on outcome [8]. The choice between monofilament and braided synthetic tape should be a personal choice based on personal preference and clinical experience.

The McDonald cerclage technique has never been directly compared by randomized clinical trial with the Shirodkar technique with respect to perinatal outcome. The Shirodkar type of cerclage has been advocated by some because of the ability to achieve a close proximity to the internal os [9]. One study has analyzed McDonald cerclage location in reference to the internal os and its influence on outcome [10]. They found that cerclage placement closer to the internal os had no discernable effect on outcome. Cerclage placement should be according to personal technical and clinical experience with respect to the limits of the maternal anatomy. Transabdominal cerclage requires an intraperitoneal incision to identify the lower uterine segment. This procedure can be associated with significantly more morbidity than the transvaginal approach. For this reason, the transabdominal approach is reserved for patients with serious demonstrable anatomic defects or a history of failed transvaginal procedures.

Elective cerclage

There have been four randomized trials of elective cerclage. Rush and colleagues in 1984 [11] from South Africa studied 194 patients at high risk for pregnancy loss randomly assigned elective McDonald cerclage or no cerclage. They found elective cerclage did not improve outcome. A French study by Lazar and colleagues [12] in 1984 analyzed 506 women with a history suspicious for pregnancy loss and randomly assigned them to elective McDonald cerclage or no cerclage. Again, there was no significant difference in pregnancy loss or preterm birth prevention by elective cerclage. In 1993, the Royal College of Obstetrics and Gynecology completed the largest study to date [13]. They studied 1292 patients with a suspicious obstetric history who were randomly assigned to elective cerclage or continued clinical evaluation. They concluded that approximately 96% of elective cerclage procedures were unnecessary and there was no improvement in overall perinatal outcome. In a post hoc analysis, those patients with three or more pregnancy losses seemed to have improved outcomes associated with cerclage. In 2000, a study from the Netherlands by Althuisus and colleagues [14] examined 70 patients with a classic history for cervical incompetence. On a one-to-two basis, they were randomly assigned to elective McDonald cerclage or urgent cerclage if indicated by ultrasound criteria. They concluded that in 59% of patients receiving elective cerclage, the procedure was unnecessary despite a classic history of cervical incompetence. There was no difference in perinatal outcome and 8.7% of their patients who received an elective cerclage developed ultrasound cervical changes later in pregnancy.

These two most recent studies [13,14] demonstrate the inability of historic criteria to define clearly those patients who are at risk for second-trimester loss and early preterm labor birth. In addition, most patients with a history consistent with the traditional diagnosis of cervical incompetence do not have recurrent pregnancy loss. The evidence to support the routine use of elective cerclage based on historic criteria is lacking even in those patients with classic risk factors for second-trimester loss. Based on the US Preventative Services Task Force ranking of evidence and recommendation (Table 2), the evidence-based level A I recommendations for elective cerclage are that high-risk patients can be followed safely with serial transvaginal ultrasound of the cervix during the second trimester and unnecessary cerclage procedures can be avoided. Because of the post hoc nature of the Royal College of Obstetrics and Gynecology data, a level B II-2 recommendation for elective cerclage placement in those patients with three or more losses can be considered [13]. Based on these recommendations, the routine use of elective cerclage for historic criteria should be discontinued in favor of serial transvaginal assessment of endocervical length. There are three exceptions to this recommendation: (1) a clear anatomic defect involving or near the internal os, (2) three or more second-trimester losses, or (3) inability to follow patients with reliable transvaginal ultrasound.

There remain some unanswered questions concerning elective cerclage and the authors' recommendations concerning these questions are based on level C-III clinical opinions derived from their experience.

Should low-risk patients be screened?

At the author's facility, those patients between 16 and 24 weeks' gestational age receiving ultrasound evaluation for reasons other than cervical measurements are screened by the transabdominal approach. Any suspected transabdominal abnormalities are then investigated with transvaginal ultrasound. It should be noted that transabdominal assessment alone of abnormalities of the cervix is insufficient for evaluation and the transvaginal approach is far superior. This recommendation is consistent with the American College of Radiology guidelines [15]. The exception to this rule is those cases with preterm premature

Table 2
US Preventative Services Task Force level of evidence and recommendation ranking

I	Evidence obtained from at least one properly designed randomized controlled trial.
II-1	Evidence obtained from well-designed controlled trials without randomization.
II-2	Evidence obtained from well-designed cohort or case-control analytic studies, preferably from more than one center or research group.
II-3	Evidence obtained from multiple time series with or without the intervention. Dramatic results in uncontrolled experiments also could be regarded as this type of evidence.
III	Opinions of respected authorities, based on clinical experience, descriptive studies, or reports of expert committees.
Level A	The recommendation is based on good and consistent scientific evidence.
Level B	The recommendation is based on limited or inconsistent scientific evidence.
Level C	The recommendation is based primarily on consensus and expert opinion.

rupture of the membranes in which foreign body placement into the vagina is relatively contraindicated (see the article by Berghella elsewhere in this issue).

How often should high-risk patients be screened?

Based on the authors' experience, any patient at risk for second-trimester loss or preterm birth should not be screened before 16 weeks' gestational age. Normal cervical parameters for the first trimester have not been established and pregnancies that end before this gestational age are usually associated with the pathophysiology of first-trimester loss, which has multiple and diverse etiologies. Between 16 and 24 weeks any patient with a significant risk factor (previous preterm birth, previous second-trimester loss, prior cervical surgery, diethyl-stilbestrol exposure, mullerian anomaly, multiple gestation, and so forth) is evaluated every 1 to 4 weeks depending on the significance of the risk factor or the presence of multiple risk factors. For example, a patient with prior cervical surgery and term delivery is followed on a monthly basis, whereas the patient with a prior second-trimester loss and cervical surgery is followed on a 1- to 2-week basis.

What should be done with high-risk patients with gross anatomic defects?

Patients with cervical lacerations that extend into the lower uterine segment or gynecologic surgical amputation are candidates for elective transabdominal cerclage. It should be noted that these patients are relatively uncommon (the authors' institutional ratio of transabdominal cerclage patients to transvaginal cerclage candidates is 1:50). These cases should be referred to those institutions with experience in treating these exceedingly high-risk patients with ab-dominal cerclage.

Urgent cerclage

The evidence supporting the use of urgent cerclage was based on sonographic findings and was supported by initial retrospective and descriptive studies [16–18]. Unfortunately, the widespread use of urgent cerclage for a shortened cervix or transvaginal ultrasound preceded extensive scientific scrutiny. In 1995, Iams and colleagues [19] documented the changes in the cervix that take place over time and are visualized by transvaginal ultrasound. They concluded that closed cervical length has a direct relationship with gestational age at birth (as cervical length decreases, the probability of term birth decreases). This con-tinuum theory is compatible with the predictable "T,Y,V,U" process originally described by Zilianti and colleagues [20]. Before the onset of dilation and effacement, the fetal membranes in the endocervical canal have a perpendicular T-shaped relationship (Fig. 1). As the cervix begins to efface, the internal os becomes disrupted, and the fetal membranes prolapse into the endocervical canal

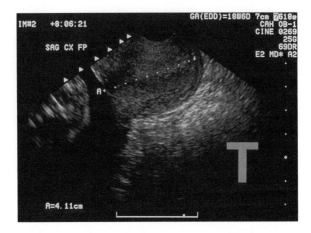

Fig. 1. Transvaginal ultrasound image of a normal-appearing cervix. Note the perpendicular "T" shape relationship between the fetal membranes and endocervical canal.

producing a funnel or Y-shaped finding on transvaginal ultrasound (Fig. 2). It should be noted that during this phase there is usually no manifestation of change noted at the level of the external os with direct vaginal speculum visualization or with digital examination. As the membranes continue to descend into the endocervical canal and the closed cervical length shortens, there can be a V shape noted on transvaginal ultrasound (Fig. 3). The classic V shape represents a brief transition from the Y to U phase and is seen much less often then these other two shapes. The characteristic U-shaped membrane prolapsed into the endocervical canal is associated with a markedly reduced cervical length and is usually associated with findings at the level of the external os including visible

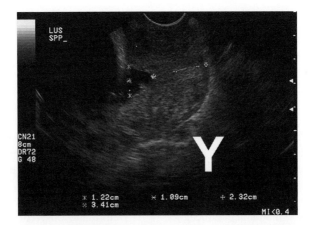

Fig. 2. Transvaginal ultrasound demonstrating the characteristic "Y" shape funnel caused by dilation of the internal os, prolapse of the fetal membranes into the endocervical canal, and a shortened distal cervical segment.

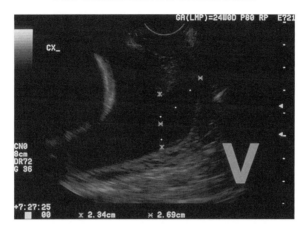

Fig. 3. Transvaginal ultrasound demonstrating further membrane prolapse and a very short distal cervical length associated with the "V" shape.

membranes on speculum examination and significant dilation or effacement noted on digital examination (Fig. 4).

The theory of the loss of cervical competence as a continuum establishes this predictable sequence of progressive cervical dilation and effacement similar to the process that normally takes place near-term. It further suggests a similar pathophysiology related to these ultrasound changes when they occur in the second trimester (loss of cervical competence) and early third trimester (preterm labor). In 1996, Iams and colleagues [21] as part of the National Institute of Health Maternal Fetal Medicine network, established a cervical length of less than or equal to 2.5 cm at 24 weeks as the 10th percentile and the critical threshold for increased risk of preterm birth. Since that time there have been four

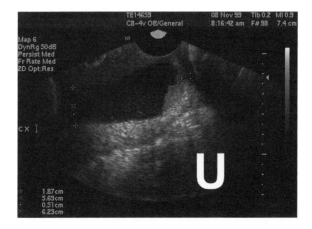

Fig. 4. Transvaginal ultrasound demonstrating the "U" shape membrane prolapse with an extremely short distal cervical segment. These ultrasound findings are usually associated with changes in the external os visible on speculum examination and palpable on digital examination.

Table 3
Efficacy of urgent cerclage

	Dutch [23]	Lehigh Valley [22,43]	Thomas Jefferson [25]	Multinational [24]
Dates of enrollment	1995–2000	1998–2003	1998–2003	Unspecified
Sample size	35	241	61	252
Historic criteria	Singleton, previous PTB (48%); gyn surgery or anomaly (23%); cervical findings only (28%)	All patients, previous PTB (42%); gyn surgery or anomaly (31%); multiple gestation (14%); cervical findings only (12%)	All patients, previous PTB or gyn factor (77%); multiple gestation (6%); cervical findings only (16%)	Singleton, previous PTB (18%); gyn factor (39%); cervical finding only (43%)
Cervical criteria	Length <2.5 cm (mean 2.0)	Length <2.5 cm with funnel (mean 1.7)	<2.5 cm with funnel (mean 1.6 cm)	<1.5 cm 94% with funnel (mean 0.9 cm)
Gest age range	Lower limit unspecified up to 27 wk (mean 20.7)	16–24 wk (mean 20.9)	14–23 (mean 19.3)	22–25 wk (mean 23.5)
Amniocentesis to rule out infection	No	Yes	No	No
Medical treatment	All patients: 6 days of metronidazole and amoxicillin; Cerclage patients: perioperative indomethacin	All patients: preoperative clindamycin and indomethacin X48–72 h then continue postoperative × 24 h	Unspecified	Cerclage patients: erythromycin one dose preoperative; All patients: steroids 26–28 wk
Suture type and technique	Single, braided tape, McDonald	Single, nonabsorbable monofilament, McDonald	Single, braided tape, McDonald	Single braided tape, Shirodkar
Mean gestational age at delivery (wk)				
Cerclage	37.9 ± 1.2	34.2 ± 5.7	32.6 ± 6.9	36.4 ± 4.7
No cerclage	33.1 ± 6.4	34.5 ± 5.2	32.9 ± 6.7	35.4 ± 5.0
Perinatal death				
Cerclage %	0	14.4	26	6
No cerclage %	18.7	7.7	13	8

Abbreviations: Gyn, gynecologic; PTB, pre-term birth.

randomized trials that have examined the efficacy of urgent cerclage [22–25]. These four studies are summarized in Table 3. Although one of these trials has demonstrated a benefit of cerclage therapy, it should be noted that this study had the smallest sample size [23]. The combined findings of these four trials coupled with the cervical competence as a continuum theory leave one to conclude the abnormal sonographic findings of the internal os, prolapse and membranes into the endocervical canal, and shortening of the distal cervix with the dynamic change noted with the application of transfundal pressure are anatomic manifestations of altered cervical physiology. Furthermore, the "T,Y,V,U" sequence noted on transvaginal ultrasound may be a final common pathway of multiple pathophysiologic processes (Fig. 5). Evidence-based level A I recommendations for urgent cerclage include the following: the group of patients who benefit from urgent cerclage has yet to be defined, urgent cerclage should be considered a procedure under investigation, and obstetric departments or divisions of maternal-fetal medicine should establish protocols for these very complex patients. The authors further recommend (level C III) that data be collected on treatment protocol results and intermittently evaluated. Harger [26] recently reviewed the literature on cerclage therapy and recommended treatment protocols for elective, urgent, and emergent cerclage. The authors consider these excellent templates for treatment protocols.

Several questions regarding urgent cerclage remain unanswered. The following suggestions are based on the authors' experience and clinical opinion, and should be considered level C III.

Other than cerclage, are there any other adjunctive treatments with antibiotics, tocolytics, or steroids that may benefit the patient?

All patients with these sonographic changes during the second trimester should have multiple urogenital cultures to rule out subclinical infection. In the authors' treatment protocols at Lehigh Valley Hospital, they included an amnio-

Final Common Pathway

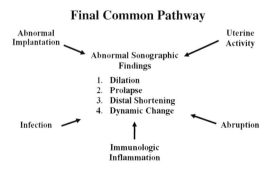

Fig. 5. A schematic diagram demonstrating some of the multiple pathophysiologic processes that may be associated with cervical changes on transvaginal ultrasound in the second trimester. (*Modified from* Rust OA, Atlas RO, Reed J, et al. Revisiting the short cervix detected by transvaginal ultrasound in the second trimester: why cerclage therapy may not help. Am J Obstet Gynecol 2001;185:1098–105.)

centesis to rule out evidence of significant intra-amniotic infection [22]. It should be noted that amniocentesis was used as part of an Institutional Review Board protocol and should not be considered for routine care. Short-course antibiotic therapy can be considered before cerclage placement or as empiric medical therapy, but it should be noted that there is no evidence to support such treatment. In addition, long-term antibiotic therapy should be avoided because of the potential for selection of resistant organisms. In the case of tocolytic therapy, the authors use short-term indomethacin for its anti-inflammatory and tocolytic effects. There are no data to support its empiric use. The absence of anti-inflammatory properties for magnesium sulfate, nifedipine, and β-agonists precludes their use in the authors' opinion. Concerning the use of corticosteroids, most of the authors' cerclage placements are before 24 weeks' gestational age. They have not used corticosteroids as part of their treatment protocol. If the patient returns, is readmitted for preterm labor, or has other significant risk factors for preterm early delivery, a single course of corticosteroids is indicated in accordance with well-established guidelines [27].

Should patients with these sonographic findings be hospitalized?

The authors recommend outpatient management of reliable patients be considered and use follow-up outpatient evaluation, at least on a weekly basis, until stabilization of endocervical length is established over a 2- to 4-week period. In the absence of a progressive decrease in the endocervical length, the intervals for evaluation can be extended to every other week. The patients should be educated as to the signs and symptoms of frequent complications including preterm labor, chorioamnionitis, and placental abruption.

After delivery, should these patients have any specific testing?

If during the pregnancy a urogenital infection is documented or there is histopathologic evidence of chorioamnionitis at the time of delivery, an evaluation for subclinical gynecologic infection is indicated. In addition, evaluation for mullerian anomalies or other alterations in the intrauterine or cervical anatomy should be considered (hysteroscopy, hysterosalpingogram, three-dimensional transvaginal ultrasound, MRI, and so forth). The patient may also benefit from preconceptual counseling with respect to the potential recurrence of sonographic findings in the second trimester.

Emergent cerclage

Emergent cerclage has been supported by multiple retrospective studies that suggest benefit [28–34]. In contrast to candidates for urgent cerclage, emergent cerclage patients have significant risk for intra-amniotic infection because of membrane exposure to the vaginal flora (Fig. 6). For this reason, before attempt-

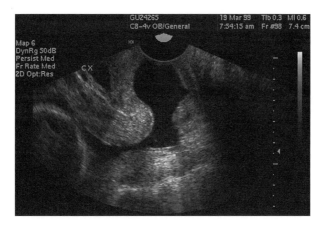

Fig. 6. Transvaginal ultrasound demonstrating membrane prolapse beyond the external os into the vaginal cavity.

ing a rescue procedure, amniocentesis should be considered. In addition, these patients should be monitored for subclinical uterine activity and the potential for placental abruption. Because of the retrospective nature of these studies, these recommendations achieve a level of B II-2. Most often, these emergent procedures represent a final effort to prevent imminent delivery of an extremely premature fetus (Fig. 7). There remain questions unanswered concerning emergent cerclage, and level C III recommendations follow.

What is the best way to reduce the membranes above the cervix before cerclage placement?

At the authors' institution a sequential method is used. First, the cervix is examined under anesthesia. If, in the Trendelenburg's position, the membranes

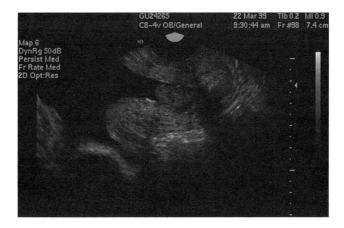

Fig. 7. Transvaginal ultrasound of the same patient in Fig. 6 post emergent cerclage.

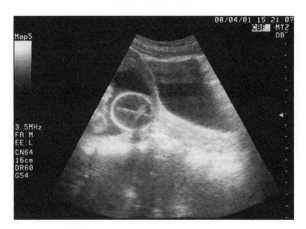

Fig. 8. A intraoperative transabdominal ultrasound demonstrating a filled bladder compressing the endocervical canal with a 16 Foley catheter with 30-mL balloon in the lower uterine segment displacing the fetal membranes above the internal os.

are at or above the external os, a 16-mL Foley catheter with 30-mL bulb is placed into the lower uterine segment and the balloon gradually filled until the membranes appear receded above the internal os by intraoperative ultrasound. With membranes persistently beyond the external os and prolapsed into the vagina, the maternal bladder is filled under ultrasound guidance to 500 to 800 mL of normal saline. If the membranes fully recede with bladder filling, then the Foley catheter is placed through the cervix and balloon inflated as described previously (Fig. 8). The bladder is then allowed to drain to facilitate cerclage placement. If bladder filling fails to reduce the membranes, then the authors consider an amniocentesis with amniotic fluid reduction to assist replacement of the membranes into the uterine cavity, and then proceed with Foley placement into the uterine cavity. The cerclage is then placed in close proximity of the internal os as possible with the suture tied as the Foley catheter balloon is drained and then removed from the cervix.

Should antibiotics or tocolytics be used?

The authors recommend a short course antibiotic and indomethacin therapy be used as described with urgent cerclage. They recommend an interval of 48 to 72 hours be used before cerclage placement to allow urogenital cultures to return and to rule out infection. In addition, the finding of membranes extended beyond the external os often is a manifestation of a rapidly progressive process for which a hastily placed cerclage may be associated with significant complication, such as cervical laceration, rapidly progressive chorioamnionitis, or precipitous preterm labor.

Should a Trendelenburg's position be used?

The use of Trendelenburg's position to enlist the help of gravity in reducing the membranes seems prudent. In the authors' experience, however, if this membrane reduction does not occur spontaneously within the first 24 hours, it most likely will not occur at all. Prolonged Trendelenburg's positioning is very uncomfortable for the patient and may increase the risk of aspiration of gastric contents. For this reason, they do not suggest Trendelenburg's positioning of longer than 24 hours.

Transabdominal cerclage

The evidence for transabdominal cerclage is also based on multiple small case series [35–37]. The evidence supporting this procedure should be considered level B II-2. The indications for a transabdominal procedure include a congenitally or surgically absent or damaged ectocervix or failed transvaginal procedures. One recent retrospective study has demonstrated that perinatal outcome seems to be improved in patients with prior failed transvaginal cerclage when using the transabdominal approach rather than repeat transvaginal approach [37]. Transabdominal cerclage is usually placed with timing similar to elective cerclage (between 10 and 14 weeks). There have been various modifications of the transabdominal cerclage procedure and these case reports and clinical opinions should be considered level C III recommendations. Transabdominal cerclage can be placed before pregnancy. There is concern, however, for cervical stenosis and infertility with this modification in timing [38]. When transabdominal cerclage is

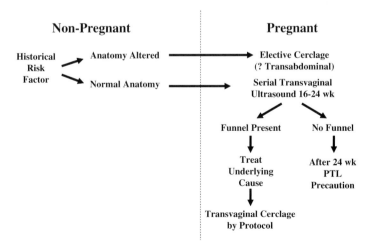

Fig. 9. The Lehigh Valley Management Protocol for patients at risk for recurrent pregnancy loss. PTL, Preterm labor precautions.

performed on an emergent basis there is considerable risk of adverse perinatal outcome. For this reason the authors recommend this procedure only be used in the most extreme circumstances and under the guidance of those surgeons with considerable experience in this procedure. Operative complications of any transabdominal procedure include preterm premature rupture of the membranes, placental abruption, stillbirth, growth restriction, preterm labor, and suture erosion or migration. For this reason, considerable counseling considering the risks versus benefits of an abdominal procedure should be used. Laparoscopic placement or cerclage removal of abdominal cerclage has also been reported [39,40]. A proposed management protocol for patients at risk for second-trimester loss is summarized in Fig. 9.

Cerclage in multifetal gestation

The use of elective cerclage in multifetal gestations has been studied by Dor and colleagues [41] in 1982. They randomly assigned 50 twin gestations to elective cerclage versus no cerclage and found no difference in outcome (level A I). Newman and colleagues [42] in a large retrospective study analyzed 128 twins comparing those pregnancies with a short cervix on transvaginal ultrasound treated with urgent cerclage with those treated without cerclage. No difference in outcome was noted (level B II-2). A recent randomized trial of urgent cerclage analyzed a subgroup of multifetal gestation patients [43]. They found that the cerclage group delivered earlier compared with the no-cerclage group (29.4 ± 5.4 weeks cerclage versus 33.1 ± 42 weeks no-cerclage, $P = .03$). Because of the analysis as a subgroup, this should be interpreted as a level B II-2 recommendation. To date, there is no evidence to support the use of elective, urgent, or emergent cerclage in multiple gestations. Considering the potential for adverse outcome, any cerclage placement in a patient with multifetal gestation should be under a research protocol and in-depth discussion with the patient of risks versus benefits used.

References

[1] Herman GE. Notes on Emmet's operation as a prevention of abortion. J Obstet Gynaecol Br Commonw 1902;2:256–7.
[2] Shirodkar VN. A new method of operative treatment for habitual abortions in the second trimester of pregnancy. Antiseptic 1955;52:299–300.
[3] McDonald IA. Suture of the cervix for inevitable miscarriage. J Obstet Gynaecol Br Commow 1957;64:346.
[4] Iams JD. Cervical incompetence. In: Creasy RK, Resnik R, editors. Maternal-fetal medicine. 4th edition. Philadelphia: WB Saunders; 1999. p. 445–64.
[5] Guzman ER, Houlihan C, Vintzileos A. Sonography and transfundal pressure in the evaluation of the cervix during pregnancy. Obstet Gynecol Surv 1995;50:395–403.
[6] Kurup M, Goldkrand JW. Cervical incompetence: elective, emergent, or urgent cerclage. Am J Obstet Gynecol 1999;181:240–6.

[7] Aarts JM, Brons JTJ, Bruinse HW. Emergency cerclage: a review. Obstet Gynecol Surv 1995;50:459–69.

[8] Pereira L, Llevy C, Lewis D, et al. Effect of suture material on the outcome of emergent cerclage. Obstet Gynecol 2004;103:35S.

[9] Novy MJ, Haymond J, Nichols M. Shirodkar cerclage in a multifactorial approach to the patient with advanced cervical changes. Am J Obstet Gynecol 1990;162:1412–9.

[10] Rust OA, Atlas RO, Meyn J, et al. Does cerclage location influence perinatal outcome? Am J Obstet Gynecol 2003;189:1688–91.

[11] Rush RW, Isaacs S, McPherson K, et al. A randomized controlled trial of cervical cerclage in women at high risk of spontaneous preterm delivery. Br J Obstet Gynaecol 1984;91:724–30.

[12] Lazar P, Guegan S. Multicentred controlled trial of cervical cerclage in women at moderate risk of preterm delivery. Br J Obstet Gynaecol 1984;91:731–5.

[13] MRC/RCOG Working Party on Cervical Cerclage. Final report of the Medical Research Council/Royal College of Obstetricians and Gynaecologists Multicentre Randomised trial of cervical cerclage. Br J Obstet Gynaecol 1993;100:516–23.

[14] Althuisius SM, Dekker GA, van Geijn HP, et al. Cervical Incompetence Prevention Randomized Cerclage Trial (CIPRACT): study design and preliminary results. Am J Obstet Gynecol 2000;183:823–9.

[15] American College of Radiology. ACR appropriateness criteria. Expert Panel on Women's Imaging. Premature cervical dilatation. Reston (VA): American College of Radiology; 1999.

[16] Guzman ER, Rosenberg JC, Houlihan C, et al. A new method using vaginal ultrasound and transfundal pressure to evaluate the asymptomatic incompetent cervix. Obstet Gynecol 1994;83:248–52.

[17] Fox R, James M, Tuohy J, et al. Transvaginal ultrasound in the management of women with suspected cervical incompetence. Br J Obstet Gynaecol 1996;103:921–4.

[18] Guzman ER, Pisatowski DM, Vintzileos AM, et al. A comparison of ultrasonographically detected cervical changes in response to transfundal pressure, coughing, and standing in predicting cervical incompetence. Am J Obstet Gynecol 1997;177:660–5.

[19] Iams JD, Johnson FF, Sonek J, et al. Cervical competence as a continuum: a study of ultrasonographic cervical length and obstetric performance. Am J Obstet Gynecol 1995;172:1097–106.

[20] Zilianti M, Azuaga A, Calderon F, et al. Monitoring the effacement of the uterine cervix by transperineal sonography: a new perspective. J Ultrasound Med 1995;14:719–24.

[21] Iams JD, Goldenberg RL, Meis PJ, et al. The length of the cervix and the risk of spontaneous premature delivery. N Engl J Med 1996;334:567–72.

[22] Rust OA, Atlas RO, Reed J, et al. Revisiting the short cervix detected by transvaginal ultrasound in the second trimester: why cerclage therapy may not help. Am J Obstet Gynecol 2001;185:1098–105.

[23] Althuisius SM, Dekker GA, Hummel P, et al. Final results of the cervical incompetence prevention randomized cerclage trial (CIPRACT): therapeutic cerclage with bed rest versus bed rest alone. Am J Obstet Gynecol 2001;185:1106–12.

[24] To MS, Alfirevic Z, Heath VCF, et al. Cervical cerclage for prevention of preterm delivery in women with short cervix: randomized controlled trial. Lancet 2004;363:1849–53.

[25] Berghella V, Odibo AO, Tolosa JE. Cerclage for prevention of preterm birth in women with a short cervix found on transvaginal examination: a randomized trial. Am J Obstet Gynecol 2004;191:1311–7.

[26] Harger JH. Cerclage and cervical insufficiency: an evidence-based analysis. Obstet Gynecol 2002;100:1313–27.

[27] American College of Obstetricians and Gynecologists. Antenatal corticosteroid therapy for fetal maturation. Committee opinion No. 273. Washington: American College of Obstetricians and Gynecologists; 2002.

[28] Novy J, Gupta A, Wothe DD, et al. Cervical cerclage in the second trimester of pregnancy: a historical cohort study. Am J Obstet Gynecol 2001;184:1447–56.

[29] Latta RA, McKenna B. Emergency cervical cerclage: predictors of success or failure. J Matern Fetal Neonatal Med 1996;5:22–7.

[30] Lipitz S, Libshitz A, Oelsner G, et al. Outcome of second-trimester emergency cervical cerclage in patients with no history of cervical incompetence. Am J Perinatol 1996;13:419–22.

[31] Mitra AG, Katz VL, Bowes Jr WL, et al. Emergency cerclages: a review of 40 consecutive procedures. Am J Perinatol 1992;9:142–5.

[32] Chasen ST, Silverman NS. Mid-trimester emergent cerclage: a ten year single institution review. J Perinatol 1998;18:338–42.

[33] Schorr SJ, Morales WJ. Obstetric management of incompetent cervix and bulging fetal membranes. J Reprod Med 1996;41:235–8.

[34] Wong GP, Farquharson DF, Dansereau J. Emergency cervical cerclage: a retrospective review of 51 cases. Am J Perinatol 1993;10:341–6.

[35] Cammarano CL, Herron MA, Parer JT. Validity of indications for transabdominal cervicoisthmic cerclage for cervical incompetence. Am J Obstet Gynecol 1995;172:1871–5.

[36] Novy MJ. Transabdominal cervicoisthmic cerclage: a reappraisal 25 years after its introduction. Am J Obstet Gynecol 1991;164:1635–42.

[37] Davis G, Berghella V, Talucci M, et al. Patients with prior failed transvaginal cerclage: a comparison of obstetric outcomes with either transabdominal or transvaginal cerclage. Am J Obstet Gynecol 2000;183:836–9.

[38] Norwitz ER, Lee DM, Goldstein DP. Transabdominal cervicoisthmic cerclage: learning to tie the knot. J Gynecol Tech 1996;2:49–54.

[39] Scarantino SE, Reilly JG, Moretti ML, et al. Laparoscopic removal of a transabdominal cervical cerclage. Am J Obstet Gynecol 2000;182:1086–8.

[40] Al-Fadhli R, Tulandi T. Laparoscopic abdominal cerclage. Clin Obstet Gynecol 2004;31:497–504.

[41] Dor J, Shaley J, Mashiach S, et al. Elective cervical suture of twin pregnancies diagnosed ultrasonically in the first trimester following induced ovulation. Gynecol Obstet Invest 1982;13:55–60.

[42] Newman RB, Krombach RS, Myers MC, et al. Effect of cerclage on obstetrical outcome in twin gestations with a shortened cervical length. Am J Obstet Gynecol 2002;186:634–40.

[43] Rust OA, Atlas RO, Fischl S, et al. The Lehigh Valley randomized trial of cerclage versus no cerclage: is there a subgroup of patients that would benefit from urgent cerclage? Am J Obstet Gynecol, 2005.

ELSEVIER
SAUNDERS

Obstet Gynecol Clin N Am
32 (2005) 457–484

OBSTETRICS AND
GYNECOLOGY
CLINICS
OF NORTH AMERICA

β-Agonist Tocolytic Therapy

Fung Lam, MD*, Pamela Gill, RN, MSN

Department of Obstetrics and Gynecology, California Pacific Medical Center, 3838 California Street, Suite 812, San Francisco, CA 94118, USA

β-Adrenergic agents have been prescribed by physicians to arrest preterm labor for more than 30 years. These medications, including terbutaline, ritodrine, isoproterenol, isoxsuprine, fenoterol, hexaprenaline, and salbutamol, enjoy a long history and worldwide use as tocolytic agents [1]. Since 1998, with the voluntary withdrawal of ritodrine by its distributor from the American market, terbutaline remains the only β-adrenergic tocolytic agent available in the United States [2]. Indeed, there currently is not a single tocolytic agent that is approved for use in pregnancy in the United States by the Food and Drug Administration (FDA).

Three decades ago, the inhibition of preterm labor was applicable to only a minority of women [3]. With the advent of preterm birth prevention programs, which emphasize patient and provider education, identify patients at risk, facilitate early diagnosis, and provide for aggressive and expeditious therapy, increasing numbers of patients are now considered candidates for tocolytic management. Tocolysis' chief benefit is significantly prolonging pregnancy in the hope of avoiding or ameliorating the sequelae of preterm delivery. Delaying delivery even a short time allows for administration of steroids and in utero transfer of mother, thereby enabling preterm infants to be delivered in obstetric units experienced in the care of high-risk pregnancies along with their supportive neonatal intensive care facilities. At early gestational ages, even a modest (48–72 hour) prolongation of pregnancy can be greatly beneficial to the fetus and improve neonatal outcomes [2]. Tocolytic prolongation of pregnancy can also be beneficial when there are underlying or self-limited causes of labor, such as pyelonephritis or abdominal surgery, that are unlikely to cause recurrent preterm labor [4,5]. The function of acute tocolysis is not necessarily to prevent a preterm delivery.

---

* Corresponding author.
E-mail address: funglamMD@aol.com (F. Lam).

Three principal indications dominate the use of tocolysis in the treatment of preterm labor: (1) prophylaxis (ie, therapy based on the presence of a risk factor or uterine activity alone, in the absence of documented cervical change, to prevent preterm labor); (2) acute therapy (ie, typically administration of parenteral agents by either the intravenous or subcutaneous route for prompt control of the acute episode of preterm labor for durations varying between 24–72 hours); and (3) maintenance (ie, the use of oral or subcutaneous medications for long-term tocolysis after cessation of preterm labor to prevent the recurrence of uterine activity) [6].

Food and Drug Administration

Historically, the only medication approved by the FDA in the United States for use as a tocolytic for preterm labor was ritodrine. Other tocolytic agents, such as terbutaline, salbutamol, fenoterol, and hexoprenaline, have been approved for use in many countries outside of the United States [1,7]. Originally approved for use in 1980, ritodrine, despite its FDA approval, was supplanted over the last 20 years by terbutaline for use as a maintenance tocolytic. Terbutaline is much less expensive than ritodrine, costing approximately 10 times less on a milligram-to-milligram basis. Terbutaline is also the only tocolytic agent that can be given subcutaneously. This route of administration is useful when labor-inhibiting concentrations are required rapidly and the intravenous route is not available or not desirable [1]. By 1993, between 8 and 10 times more terbutaline was used in the United States for a pregnancy-related diagnosis than the FDA-approved drug ritodrine. In the face of a diminishing market and increased regulatory pressure, the manufacturer voluntarily withdrew ritodrine from the market (first oral ritodrine in 1993 and then the intravenous injection in 1998) [2].

Terbutaline is currently FDA-approved only for the treatment of asthma, but off-label use of terbutaline as a tocolytic agent has been known to clinicians for more than 30 years. As a result of physician acceptance and comfort in prescribing terbutaline, it is now estimated that at least 260,000 women per year receive terbutaline during pregnancy and that it is the most commonly prescribed β-adrenergic for tocolysis [1,2,7,8]. In addition to its use in preterm labor, terbutaline is frequently used to effect uterine relaxation in external version for breech presentations and for rescue tocolysis for uterine tetany (in preterm and term labor). Clinicians have also used subcutaneous terbutaline to differentiate between true and false preterm labor. Since 1993, the FDA has followed its long-standing policy on the use of approved drugs for nonlabeled indications as being entirely appropriate on the basis of medical advances reported in the literature [2,6,9]. Indeed, in 1993 the FDA expressed the possibility of a literature-only based new-drug application from the manufacturer for approval for use as a tocolytic [2]. Unfortunately, no manufacturer has made this submission to the FDA. Accordingly, many tocolytic drugs have never been approved for preterm labor, but obstetricians use them because they know the drugs work [9]. FDA approval may lag behind the medical literature and current practice. To receive approval, a pharmaceutical company must demonstrate that the medication is both safe and effective in treating a certain condition. Even when the approved drug is widely used to treat other conditions, a drug maker may decide it is not cost effective to pursue supplemental approvals, so these costs may reach hundreds of millions of dollars. The company may also elect not to seek additional FDA approvals because it does not want to expose itself to potential liability [9]. For example, the manufacturer of terbutaline issues a package insert that states "parenteral terbutaline is not indicated for tocolysis" [1]. Currently approved FDA labeling for terbutaline contains warnings or precautions against use in preterm labor that are not found outside the United States.

On November 13, 1997, the FDA issued a "Dear Colleague" letter stating concerns about the subcutaneous administration of terbutaline for the treatment and prevention of preterm labor. This action seemed to have been prompted by adverse anecdotal reports. Subsequent published reports in large treated populations demonstrate that the overall incidence of severe adverse events in women treated with subcutaneous terbutaline was low and the therapy was well tolerated. The reported safety and efficacy parameters were well within the guidelines established by the previous FDA-approved β-adrenergic agent, ritodrine [9].

Physiology

β-Adrenergic agents stimulate the β-adrenergic receptors of the sympathetic nervous system. Interactions with the receptor sites cause an increase in intracellular production of cyclic adenosine monophosphate. This phenomenon results in the reduction of intracellular calcium concentration in the smooth muscle. The lower level of calcium inhibits activation of the contractile proteins actin and myosin, which in turn results in relaxation of the myometrium. Two types of β-receptors exist: β_1 and β_2 (Box 1). Because terbutaline possess β_2-specific properties, it is the drug of choice when uterine relaxation is desired. Box 2 lists the major adverse effects from β_1 stimulation. With prolonged or high-dose exposure to β-adrenergic therapy, there is a reduced response (of both end-target and peripheral cells) thought to be caused by down-regulation of the β-receptors [10–15]. Clinically, this tachyphylaxis phenomenon may be a factor in recurrent preterm labor despite treatment [16].

Studies into patterns of uterine activity have yielded valuable physiologic data. Low-amplitude high-frequency uterine activity (LAHF) is thought by many to be the precursor of more organized, phasic contractions that lead to cervical change and preterm delivery. Current investigations address the following issues: (1) can the detection of increased LAHF uterine activity be used as a screening tool to diagnose preterm labor at an earlier stage, (2) can LAHF contractions be suppressed with tocolytic agents, and (3) can suppression of this activity be achieved with smaller doses of tocolytic agents? [16–27].

Box 1. Receptor stimulation by β-adrenergic agents

β₁-Receptor

    Heart rate increased
    Heart force increased
    Lipolysis increased
    Intestinal motility decreased

β₂-Receptor

    Uterine relaxation
    Arteriole relaxation
    Bronchiole relaxation
    Muscle and liver stimulation: glycogenolysis
    Pancreas stimulation: hyperinsulinism
    Cell stimulation: hypokalemia

A circadian pattern of uterine activity has been identified. There seems to be a nocturnal distribution of organized contractions, with 80% of all uterine activity occurring during a 6-hour peak period in the late evening. The appearance of increased LAHF activity generally preceded the onset of organized contractions. The existence of this circadian pattern of uterine activity suggests that treatment of preterm labor must be individualized. The tocolytic dose can be increased during the nocturnal peak period of uterine activity and decreased during periods of uterine quiescence. Such patient-specific regimens not only reduce overall medication requirements but also minimize the risk of tachyphylaxis and toxicity [16,28–31].

Efficacy

The use of β-adrenergic drugs for prophylaxis in twin gestations has been shown to be of no benefit [32]. Double-blinded randomized studies using placebo controls have evaluated oral fenoterol [33], terbutaline [34], and ritodrine [35,36]. All trials failed to demonstrate a significant increase in the length of gestation or increased birthweight in the treated patients. Prophylactic use in at-risk singleton gestations has not been evaluated.

The effectiveness of the different β-adrenergic drugs used clinically for acute tocolysis is comparable [1,3]. Placebo-controlled studies have demonstrated that in women with intact membranes, β-adrenergic therapy is significantly superior to placebo in prolonging pregnancy, increasing birthweight, and reducing the incidence of hyaline membrane disease [3,7]. Despite the prolongation of

Box 2. Side-effects of β-adrenergic agents

Maternal: minor

  Nausea and vomiting
  Tremors
  Anxiety
  Flushing
  Headache
  Palpitations
  Heartburn
  Constipation

Maternal: major

  Angina
  Dyspnea
  Pulmonary edema
  Myocardia ischemia
  Cardiac arrhythmias
  Myocardia infarction
  Ileus
  Hyperglycemia
  Hyperinsulinism
  Ketosis
  Hypokalemia

Fetal

  Tachycardia

Neonatal

  Hypoglycemia
  Hyperinsulinism
  Hypocalcemia
  Ketoacidosis
  Ileus

pregnancy, these studies have failed to demonstrate a significant reduction in perinatal morbidity and mortality [4,37].

Overall, these studies demonstrate that acute use of these agents has the ability to inhibit uterine activity rapidly and delay delivery for 3 to 7 days, but without proved benefit to the neonate [1,4,37]. These studies were limited by small sample size, inclusion of patients with ruptured membranes, late gestational age, and inconsistent application of antenatal corticosteroids [1,4,5].

The usefulness of administering a labor-inhibiting agent for maintenance after successful suppression of an acute episode is controversial. Preliminary published data suggest that oral magnesium salts, calcium channel blockers, and prostaglandin-inhibiting agents are not effective in preventing preterm birth or prolonging pregnancy [38,39]. There is evidence, albeit weak because of sample size issues, that maintenance therapy with β-adrenergic receptor agonists can reduce the number of preterm labor recurrences and extend the time to a recurrence [40]. Subsequent meta-analysis of oral agents failed to demonstrate any improvement in outcome [41,42]. Despite this controversy, most clinicians in the United States continue to transition preterm labor patients who are stable after treatment to an oral or subcutaneous tocolytic agent for long-term maintenance until either term gestation is reached or recurrent preterm labor occurs. In this scenario, the additional goal of maintenance tocolysis becomes the detection and prevention of recurrent preterm labor and further prolongation of pregnancy [6].

Choice of β-adrenergic medication

Ritodrine was approved for use in preterm labor in 1980. During the ensuing 25 years, no other drug has been approved for use as a tocolytic by the FDA. Oral ritodrine for maintenance therapy was removed in 1993 from the United States market after the presentation of the Canadian Ritodrine trial [43]. Parenteral ritodrine has since also been removed (1998).

Terbutaline quickly supplanted ritodrine for the oral suppression of preterm labor for several reasons. First, studies showed no difference in efficacy between oral terbutaline and ritodrine. Second, the 3- to 4-hour interval dosing for terbutaline was better tolerated than the 2- to 3-hour dosing regimen for ritodrine. Finally, as a generic drug, terbutaline was much more economical than the patent-protected ritodrine. Because parenteral ritodrine was removed in 1998 and since intravenous magnesium sulfate ($MgSO_4$) was better tolerated than intravenous ritodrine at lower cost, $MgSO_4$ has become the most commonly used intravenous agent for acute tocolysis [44–48].

Maternal effects

Although designed to be specific for β_2 receptors, β-adrenergic receptor agonists affect multiple organs because of the ubiquitous nature of the β-adrenergic receptor and cross-reactivity of β_1 and β_2 receptors. Maternal cardiovascular and metabolic physiology can be significantly altered. Stimulation of the β_1 receptor increases maternal heart rate and stroke volume. Stimulation of β_2 receptors causes peripheral vasodilation and diastolic hypotension [1,4,5]. The most common cardiovascular side effects are flushing, tachycardia, palpitations, and hypotension. The most common serious side effect is pulmonary edema [1,5]. Predisposing factors include multifetal gestation; persistent tachycardia (>130 beats per minute); anemia (<9 g/dL); maternal infection; and iatrogenic fluid overload (Fig. 1) [38]. Cessation of β-adrenergic treatment and prompt diuretic treatment usually results in rapid improvement. Left untreated, adult respiratory distress syndrome can result [4]. Clinicians should pay meticulous attention to cumulative fluid intake and urine output, and perform serial pulmonary examinations. Other serious side effects can include cardiac arrhythmias, chest pain, and EKG changes. Myocardial ischemia has been reported with the severity related to high heart rates (>130 beats per minute). Known or suspected cardiac disease is a contraindication to β-adrenergic tocolysis. In addition, a prudent approach is one in which intravenous saline solutions are avoided; intravenous fluids are limited (1–2 L/d); and prolonged high-dose therapy is avoided.

Metabolic effects of the β-adrenergic tocolytics include an increase in hepatic glycogenolysis, maternal hyperglycemia, and transient hypokalemia [3,5]. Alterations in carbohydrate metabolism make other non–β-adrenergic tocolytic agents (ie, $MgSO_4$, nifedipine) more suitable for use in patients with diabetes mellitus [49]. The chronotropic effects of β-adrenergic agents may exacerbate the tachycardia associated with poorly controlled hyperthyroidism. Individualization of tocolytic therapy is critical for success and for preventing complications. The misuse of these drugs pharmacologically has, in large part, contributed to many side effects and to an apparent lack of efficacy reported by some [1]. This may also explain some of the negative efficacy reports of studies wherein a rigid protocol rather than individualization of treatment is followed.

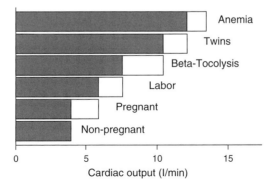

Fig. 1. Components of preterm labor and their contribution to increase in maternal cardiac output (liter per minute). (*From* Blickstein I. Maternal mortality. In: Blickstein I, Keith LG, editors. Multiple pregnancy: epidemiology, gestation and perinatal outcome. London: Taylor & Francis; 2005. p. 492–9; with permission.)

Fetal and neonatal effects

β-Adrenergic agonists freely cross the placenta and equivalent fetal serum concentrations are reached [6]. Labor-inhibiting serum concentrations of terbutaline range from 5 to 15 ng/mL. Peak plasma concentrations for terbutaline have been reported to be 12 to 31 ng/mL after intravenous infusion, 2 to 6 ng/mL for a basal subcutaneous infusion, 6 to 13 ng/mL for a 0.25-mg subcutaneous bolus, and 4 to 5 ng/mL after a 5-mg oral dose [1,6]. Direct fetal effects may include tachycardia and other physiologic and metabolic effects similar to those seen in the mother [1]. Uterine blood flow, umbilical blood flow, fetal acid-base status, and Apgar scores are not adversely affected [1,5]. Neonatal hypoglycemia, hypocalcemia, ileus, and hypotension have also been reported [4]. Transient cardiac intraventricular septal hypertrophy with ECG changes has been reported in one echocardiographic study. This effect was related to duration of exposure, was absent at follow-up, and significant lasting effects have not been substantiated [1,4,5]. The incidence of neurologic intraventricular hemorrhage is controversial. Most reviews have suggested that β-adrenergic agonists use decreased or did not affect the risk of intraventricular hemorrhage [50–53], whereas an increased risk was found in two reports [54,55]. Evaluation of children exposed to β-adrenergic agonists in utero has demonstrated that treatment does not adversely affect neurologic condition, or behavioral or psychologic development [1]. Follow-up studies of children treated in utero showed no adverse alterations at 2 years of age and at 6 years after exposure [56].

Recently, a basic science study of the effects of terbutaline in an animal model has raised some concern [57,58]. The purpose of this study of 24 rats and their litters was to examine the effects of terbutaline given on postnatal days 2 to 5 followed by exposure to insecticide on postnatal days 11 to 14 in the rat offspring. The authors reported that the insecticide alone, terbutaline alone, or the combination of both produced histologic changes in the rat brain. No long-term effect on the rat neurologic or behavioral systems was performed. The rat newborns were given terbutaline injections of 10 mg/kg/d. This is the human equivalent of 700 mg/d, 23-fold the typical oral dose (30 mg/d) given humans and 233 times the typical daily subcutaneous dose (3 mg/d). Clearly, data from these animal studies cannot convincingly link toxic effects of β-adrenergics on the developing fetus. Terbutaline is an FDA category B drug, whereas other tocolytics like nifedipine (category C) and indomethacin have no published long-term fetal safety data [59–66].

Therapeutic plan

As currently practiced, acute preterm labor (excessive uterine activity with cervical change) is promptly treated with parental tocolytics. Intravenous terbutaline is rarely used because of unacceptable side effects compared with intravenous magnesium [3,6], and intravenous ritodrine is no longer available. If acute treatment with β-adrenergic therapy for acute-onset preterm labor is contemplated, baseline evaluation should include vital signs; electronic monitoring of the fetal heart rate and uterine activity pattern; laboratory assessment (complete blood count, blood glucose, electrolytes, urinalysis with culture and sensitivity, and cervical culture); thorough pulmonary auscultation; and an EKG in patients with known or suspected cardiac conditions [67].

Initial therapy may consist only of a fluid bolus (500 mL of isotonic crystalloid over 30 minutes) administered by an indwelling line (18 gauge). If hydration is unsuccessful, therapy with subcutaneous terbutaline can be started. Terbutaline, 0.25 mg, may be given subcutaneously every 1 to 6 hours and is determined by maternal uterine activity and limited by maternal heart rate ($P > 130$ beats per minute). Subcutaneous terbutaline may be used as the primary route of administration, or it may be used to transition to maintenance therapy. Subcutaneously administered terbutaline is particularly useful when labor-inhibiting concentrations are required rapidly and the intravenous route is not available or is not desirable [1]. Presently, there is no alternative drug for this purpose. If a repeated dose of subcutaneous terbutaline is unsuccessful in achieving uterine quiescence for acute preterm labor, an alternative tocolytic agent (ie, intravenous $MgSO_4$) should be quickly initiated.

Patients at highest risk for pulmonary edema include women with multiple gestations, those with fluid overload, or women with underlying infection. Initial symptoms may include shortness of breath, coughing, or wheezing [1,5,6]. Maximum fluid administration should not exceed 2000 mL per 24 hours. Monitoring of intake and output must be strictly maintained. Oral fluid intake should also be monitored, and a positive fluid balance should be avoided. Patients should be weighed daily. The monitoring of metabolic status during therapy includes repeated evaluations of glucose levels, complete blood count, and electrolyte status.

After successful treatment, patients with preterm labor can be discharged home on oral maintenance β-adrenergic therapy. The potential advantages of oral therapy at home include reduced risks, reduced costs, decreased stress, and ease of administration [67]. Prevention of recurrent preterm labor is the goal of long-term tocolysis. During episodes of recurrent preterm labor, patients are at risk for premature rupture of membranes, further cervical change, and preterm delivery. Among the many potential causes of tocolytic failure are patient noncompliance, drug-side effects, premature rupture of membranes, and the emergence of drug tolerance. In addition, oral medications are poorly absorbed during pregnancy [68–70]. For all these reasons, many clinicians transition patients to terbutaline (discussed later).

Subcutaneous pump therapy

Subcutaneous pump therapy was developed as an alternative to intravenous tocolysis in patients who failed oral treatment because of recurrent preterm labor

[16]. Subcutaneous pump therapy delivers a continuous low basal rate of terbutaline and scheduled boluses of 0.25 mg of this agent during identified periods of increased uterine activity. The total average daily dose (including basal and bolus infusions) is 3 to 4 mg/d, and this dose is titrated according to changes in uterine activity. Resensitization of the β-receptors is essential to the success of this therapy. Patients are first maintained on intravenous $MgSO_4$ for 24 to 48 hours as a drug holiday to allow the β-receptors to regain their sensitivity. Patients who could not otherwise be discharged to home care because of inadequate response to oral therapy may be maintained successfully on pump therapy. Nursing care plays a significant role in patient education before discharge and in the subsequent management of pump therapy in the home [68–70].

Basal infusion rates should be adjusted to minimize periods of LAHF. Dose response studies demonstrated that continuous basal terbutaline infusion rates of 0.05 to 0.08 mg/h are most effective in suppressing LAHF waves and subsequent uterine contractions. In multifetal gestations, basal infusion rates of 0.06 to 0.09 mg/h may be required, because of the higher maternal blood volume. Higher basal infusion rates should be avoided, not only because they result in more medication than necessary to control LAHF waves, but also because they fail to provide significant additional suppression of organized uterine contractions.

Bolus schedules are determined according to the patient's individual contraction pattern. Bolus doses of 0.25 to 0.30 mg are given to suppress organized uterine contractions. They are scheduled every 2 to 4 hours during the established peak period of uterine activity, and less frequently during the periods of minimal uterine activity. The typical patient requires six to eight bolus doses over a 24-hour period, resulting in a total infusion of less than 4 mg/d [16,31]. This dose level is much lower than the typical oral terbutaline dosages of 40 to 60 mg/d and typical intravenous terbutaline dosages of 60 to 80 mg/d, and minimizes complications and tachyphylaxis.

The authors start most of their patients with stabilized recurrent preterm labor on a standard dosage schedule: a basal infusion of 0.05 mg/h and boluses of 0.25 mg at 9:00 AM, 12 noon, 3 PM, 6 PM, 8 PM, and 10 PM [16]. Patients are instructed to use supplemental demand boluses if they experience more than four to six contractions per hour, and to record them on their preterm labor log. Demand bolus histories are of value in making adjustments to the patient's routine bolus schedule. Boluses should not be given if the maternal pulse rate is greater than 110 beats per minute, and in any case, no more frequently than every hour. Whereas the currently accepted practice for titrating dosage levels of oral β-adrenergic agents relies on measuring maternal tachycardia (a secondary $β_1$ cardiac effect), patient-specific dosing with the terbutaline pump is directed toward reduction of uterine activity (a direct $β_2$ end organ effect) [23].

The schedule of intermittent boluses can be adjusted if the patient's pattern of uterine activity changes, either during the hospital stay or after discharge home. Adjustments may include increasing the frequency of boluses, adding additional boluses, increasing the individual bolus doses up to a maximum of 0.3 mg, or shifting the cluster of boluses to coincide with a shift in the period of peak uterine activity [6,16,31,67]. The basal infusion rate may be increased if there is an increase in uterine LAHF waves or a persistent increase in uterine contractions of greater than four to six per hour despite repeated boluses. It is best to maintain the basal infusion at the lowest rate possible, however, to prevent β_2 receptor site desensitization. When the patient is stable on terbutaline pump therapy, she can be discharged home on bed rest and monitored several hours per day with a portable tocodynamometer [6]. Monitoring is scheduled for 1 hour during the peak period of contractions, and 1 hour during the quiet period to determine LAHF wave activity. Additional monitoring may be needed if periods of increased uterine activity occur. A home care perinatal nurse should visit the patient on a weekly basis to check blood pressure, pulse rate, fundal height, and fetal heart rate; perform a urinalysis; and perform cervical examinations as indicated [68].

Studies of recurrent preterm labor in patients with singleton or multiple pregnancies who are receiving β-adrenergic therapy demonstrate the following patterns (Fig. 2): (1) a return of excessive levels of LAHF contractions; (2) a return of a circadian, generally nocturnal, pattern of organized high-amplitude uterine contractions; (3) a rapidly increasing need for increased frequency and dosing of terbutaline or ritodrine [6,67]; and (4) a crescendo effect or acceleration of the frequency of uterine contractions 48 to 72 hours before the episode of active recurrent preterm labor [71]. Studies have shown that the home uterine activity monitor is useful in titrating tocolysis at home and reducing unnecessary hospital admissions unless they are required to institute or reinstitute intravenous tocolysis [24,25,27,28]. Although infrequent, breakthrough does occur in patients receiving terbutaline pump therapy. If it does, the patient should be readmitted to the hospital and stabilized on intravenous $MgSO_4$ for 24 to 48 hours. Terbutaline pump therapy should be discontinued (both basal and bolus infusions). This drug

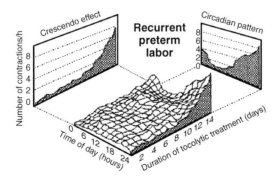

Fig. 2. Three-dimensional plot of uterine activity in a twin gestation leading to recurrent preterm labor: continuous monitoring of a patient on oral terbutaline therapy. Recurrent preterm labor is characterized by (1) a return of excessive levels of low-amplitude, high-frequency precursor uterine activity patterns; (2) a return of a circadian, generally nocturnal pattern of organized high-amplitude uterine contractions; (3) a rapidly increasing need for increased frequency and dosage of terbutaline; and (4) a crescendo effect of acceleration of frequency of uterine contractions 48 to 72 hours before the episode of active recurrent preterm labor.

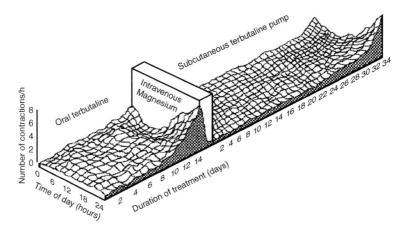

Fig. 3. Recurrent preterm labor may be secondary to down-regulation of the uterine β-receptors. Intravenous magnesium sulfate is initiated in a sequential fashion to provide a "drug holiday." At least 24 to 48 hours is required for the uterine β-receptors to up-regulate and regain their sensitivity to terbutaline. At this point, subcutaneous terbutaline pump therapy can be started to prevent the recurrence of preterm labor.

holiday allows the myometrial receptors to regain their sensitivity to terbutaline (Fig. 3) [6].

Perhaps the major cause of recurrent preterm labor is the desensitization of myometrial B_2-adrenergic receptor sites by prolonged and continuous exposure to high-dose oral β-adrenergic agents. This down-regulation phenomenon may also explain the failure of β-adrenergic tocolytics for the prophylactic treatment of preterm labor [10–16]. If the diagnosis of recurrent preterm labor is made before advanced cervical dilation (>3 cm), acute tocolysis is successful in 90% of cases if a sequential approach is taken [44]. Patients in preterm labor with tocolytic breakthrough from a β-agonist should be treated with $MgSO_4$. Because $MgSO_4$ acts differently than the β-adrenergic agents, a β-adrenergic free period allows the myometrial receptor sites to recover their sensitivity [13,16]. Patients who are treated with a β-adrenergic agent after a β-adrenergic failure have less than a 25% chance of success [44]. The minimum period for this drug holiday is 24 to 48 hours; once stable, the patient again can be considered a candidate for ambulatory tocolysis [6,16]. When stable, the patient can be restarted on terbutaline pump therapy and discharged home, with such tocolytic therapy being generally discontinued at 36 to 37 weeks.

Evidence from clinical studies using the subcutaneous terbutaline pump

Efficacy

In 1988, the authors described their initial experience using a microinfusion pump to administer a low-dose basal rate and scheduled bolus doses of subcutaneous terbutaline on nine women with recurrent preterm labor [16]. Preg-nancies were prolonged an average of 9.2 ± 4.3 weeks in this population. In a randomized fashion, they later reported on 69 patients who received either continuous subcutaneous terbutaline or oral terbutaline, following stabilization with intravenous tocolysis. In this study, those receiving subcutaneous terbutaline had their pregnancies prolonged a mean of 8.6 weeks compared with a mean of 2.4 weeks in the oral terbutaline group [72].

Other investigators have also compared continuous subcutaneous terbuta-line with oral terbutaline for ongoing tocolysis following recurrent preterm labor. In a matched-study design, Allbert and coworkers [73] compared 32 pa-tients who received subcutaneous terbutaline infusion with 32 patients who received oral therapy. When singleton and multiple gestations were combined, women achieved 72% of desired prolongation with oral therapy compared with 86% desired prolongation among those receiving subcutaneous therapy ($P < .01$). A descriptive analysis of 992 high-risk patients, including 206 twin preg-nancies receiving continuous subcutaneous terbutaline infusion, also reported by Allbert and coworkers [74], showed a mean pregnancy prolongation of 38 ± 23 days.

Adkins and colleagues [75] reported on 51 patients with preterm labor (including four with twins) who received subcutaneous terbutaline therapy after stabilization with intravenous $MgSO_4$. Subcutaneous administration of terbuta-line was successful in 98% of patients, prolonging pregnancy a mean of 6.6 weeks. Mean gestational age at delivery was 37 weeks and the mean infant birth weight was 3035 g with 85% of neonates weighing >2500 g. Only 22% of in-fants went to the neonatal ICU, with a mean stay of 7 days. Three patients reported adverse effects and had their bolus dosages decreased. No serious ad-verse events were reported.

In 1998, Lam and colleagues [76] reported on the efficacy of subcutaneous terbutaline infusion therapy in 256 singleton pregnancies with recurrent pre-term labor while on oral terbutaline. Pregnancy prolongation was found to be greater for subcutaneous versus oral administration of terbutaline (4.4 versus 2.7 weeks). The pregnancy prolongation index for subcutaneous therapy was 74% compared with 31% for oral therapy. In a similar fashion, Lam and col-leagues [77] reported on 386 women with twin gestations in preterm labor who were treated with oral terbutaline versus a like number who used subcutaneous pump therapy. Those treated with parenteral therapy in the home gained significantly more days in utero (34 ± 19.8 versus 19.3 ± 15.3 days) with a higher pregnancy prolongation index (79% versus 33% $P < .001$). Patients gained a mean of 53.4 ± 21.4 days overall with a mean gestational age at delivery of 35.2 ± 1.9 weeks. These women gained 2.8 weeks with oral terbutaline and 4.9 weeks with subcutaneous terbutaline prescribed sequentially.

Elliot and Radin [78] reported on subcutaneous terbutaline infusion therapy use in higher-order multiple gestations. Fifteen triplet and six quadruplet preg-nancies were treated with individualized dosing protocols. Triplet patients re-mained on infusion therapy for 58 days and delivered at a mean gestational age of 33 weeks. Quadruplet patients were on subcutaneous infusion therapy for 77 days and delivered at a mean gestational age of 33 weeks. Only 2 (13%) of 15 triplets and 1 (17%) of 6 quadruplets were delivered because of tocolytic failure. No one in the study had subcutaneous terbutaline discontinued because of side effects.

Angel and colleagues [79] described a clinical protocol where triplets and quadruplet pregnancies underwent a transition to subcutaneous terbutaline after intravenous $MgSO_4$ treatment for the first episode of preterm labor. Overall, 87% (20) of women with triplet gestations experienced preterm labor. The mean gestational age at delivery for triplets was 32.3 ± 0.5 weeks.

Elliot and colleagues [80] assessed the gestational gain in triplet pregnancies treated with oral terbutaline followed by continuous subcutaneous terbutaline therapy. One hundred and four triplet pregnancies were studied. The mean gestational age at enrollment was 22 ± 2.7 weeks. The study showed that these pregnancies were prolonged 52% longer (mean 5.4 ± 3.4 versus 2.8 ± 2.2 weeks) when terbutaline was administered by continuous subcutaneous infusion compared with oral administration. Overall, patients gained a mean of 8.2 ± 3.1 weeks' gestation with oral and subcutaneous terbutaline. The mean gestational age at delivery was 33.2 ± 2.2 weeks. The authors concluded that in women with triplet gestation, greater pregnancy prolongation was achieved with subcutaneous administration than with oral administration of terbutaline.

Morrison and colleagues [81] compared 15 women with singleton pregnancies and recurrent preterm labor at less than 32 weeks' gestation and treated with subcutaneous pump therapy with 45 matched control patients (3:1) treated with no tocolytic therapy after hospitalization. Gestational age at delivery more than 37 weeks (53% versus 4%), percentage delivered at less than 32 weeks overall (0% versus 47%), and pregnancy prolongation (49.8 ± 19.2 days versus 24.5 ± 12.8 days) were all significantly better in the study group. The total number of maternal hospital days, duration of neonatal ICU stay, and the total cost for newborn care favored the subcutaneous pump therapy patients. The authors concluded from this small study that the use of subcutaneous pump therapy significantly prolongs pregnancy, decreases serious neonatal complications, and reduces the duration of hospitalization for both mother and infant, and neonatal costs. When newborn hospital costs were considered, there was a much greater expenditure among the control group subjects ($62,033 \pm $89,978) compared with treated patients ($6995 \pm $14,822, $P \le .0002$). Indeed, for every dollar spent on subcutaneous pump therapy, there was a savings of $4.67 in newborn hospital costs for control patients.

Not all studies have found improved efficacy with subcutaneous pump therapy. Wenstrom and coworkers [82] enrolled 42 patients during a 4-year period having the diagnosis of preterm labor to evaluate subcutaneous infusion therapy. In this three-arm study, patients were randomized to receive either oral terbutaline, subcutaneous terbutaline infusion, or subcutaneous saline infusion. Subcutaneous drug therapy was not adjusted for patient weight or volume of distribution. Electronic home uterine contraction monitoring and daily nursing care were not used. Terbutaline boluses were adjusted for patient-reported contractions or on a rigid predetermined scale. Patients received a mean of 1.5 ± 2.4 scheduled boluses per day in the terbutaline–subcutaneous infusion group, which is considerably less than standard practice. All patients in the Wenstrom study were administered a basal rate of 0.05 mg/h, which was not titrated to the level of uterine irritability, as is customary. Patients were permitted to cross over between treatment arms if initial therapy failed. This study parameter resulted in 25% of the women initially enrolled in the placebo-saline group ultimately receiving subcutaneous terbutaline but outcomes for patients were compared only with the treatment group to which patients were originally assigned. Even with the unblinding of the assigned treatment group, the authors concluded that the three interventions were equally efficacious.

Guinn and colleagues [83] reported on 52 women randomized to either terbutaline or placebo by subcutaneous infusion. Patients did not receive daily nursing contact or home uterine activity monitoring, as is generally prescribed in obstetric practice for women receiving continuous subcutaneous terbutaline infusion in the home setting. In one half of the participants, the cervix was 3 cm or more dilated and at least 50% effaced at enrollment. Patients were enrolled at a mean of 31 weeks and were not treated for recurrent preterm labor occurring at or beyond 34 weeks, which made the hypothesized 6-week prolongation for the treatment group unlikely. Tocolytic dosing was not individualized or titrated to uterine activity, and the bolus schedule used in the study allowed a 7-hour lapse during nighttime, a period during which most stronger contractions occur [25,81]. Using this protocol, the authors reported only a 1-day difference in pregnancy prolongation between the group, with the subcutaneous terbutaline group achieving a 28.8 ± 22 day prolongation.

It is apparent that monitoring uterine activity to adjust bolus terbutaline therapy is fundamentally important. In the two negative studies, which enrolled a total of 94 women (<1% of all terbutaline pump patients reported), several methodologic flaws were likely responsible for the lack of efficacy compared with the other 37 studies in the literature [25]. First, in these studies uterine contraction monitoring and daily nursing contact were not used in either group; the bolus therapy could not be tailored for the patient. Second, pharmacy consultation was not used, so terbutaline doses were similar regardless of the weight or volume of distribution of the patients [81]. Patients in the control group of one study were switched to the terbutaline pump if oral therapy failed, but they were kept in the original group assignment for analysis [72]. In the other study [73], there was advanced cervical change (>3 cm dilated or 50% effacement) more often in the pump group at the start of the therapy. Overall, both studies had a high dropout rate (more than one third) and were significantly underpowered (>300 patients in each group were needed) [25,81]. It is important to use the subcutaneous pump therapy appropriately if clinicians are to obtain effective results in prolonging pregnancy.

Table 1
Evidence-based medicine and continuous subcutaneous terbutaline infusion: review of efficacy literature

Study	Research design	Quality of evidence	N	Population	Comments
Lam et al [89]	Observational cohort	II-2	1556	RPTL	Inclusion criterion: tocolytic breakthrough in high-risk population subset. Results: PTD rate was reduced from 5.18%–2.69% ($P < .05$)
Lam et al [16]	Descriptive case series	III	9	RPTL	Pregnancy prolongation 9.2 wk, mean GAD 39 wk.
Lam et al [72]	Randomized controlled trial	I	68	CPTL	Weeks of pregnancy prolongation and PPI were 8.6 (0.93) and 2.4 (0.34) in the pump versus oral groups, respectively.
Gianopoulos et al [90]	Descriptive case series	III	31	RPTL	Pregnancy prolongation 5.4 ± 4.5 wk and 34.2 ± 3.8 wk gestational age at delivery.
Jones et al [91]	Descriptive case series	III	50	RPTL	Pregnancy prolongation 6.3 wk.
Fischer et al [92]	Descriptive case series	III	19	CPTL	Safe and effective in the treatment of preterm labor. Average GAD 35.6 wk.
McGettigan et al [93]	Observational cohort	II-2	28	RPTL	Average GAD 35.7 wk. Terbutaline pump prolongs tocolysis, reduces terbutaline dose significantly ($P < .001$), reduces maternal side effects, and may reduce the newborn's total exposure to β-mimetic dosage.
Wolfsen and Winn [110]	Descriptive case series	III	9	Twins with advanced cervical dilatation	75% achieved >37 wk or mature lung indices on amniocentesis.
Albert et al [74]	Descriptive case series	III	992	CPTL and RPTL 206 twins 786 singletons	Extended the gestation a mean of 38 ± 23 d and average GAD 36.3 ± 2.6 wk.
Lindenbaum et al [94]	Observational cohort	II-2	725	CPTL	The incidence of gestational diabetes is not increased in patients receiving terbutaline by the subcutaneous pump.
Moise et al [95]	Descriptive case series	III	13	RPTL 10 singletons 2 triplets 1 twin	Average GAD 35.3 wk, pregnancy prolongation 5 wk.
Weinbaum et al [96]	Descriptive case series	III	202	CPTL	Contractions were arrested and the mean gestational age at delivery was 36.2 wk. Only 9.6% of the patients were readmitted to the hospital.

Study	Study design	Level of evidence	n	Condition	Comments
Elliott et al [78]	Observational case control	II-2	67	CPTL 67 quadruplets	Mean GAD 32.5 wk. Mean infant birth weight 1534 ± 429 g.
Adkins et al [75]	Descriptive case series	III	51	CPTL	Average birth weight 3000 g. Average GAD 37 wk. Pregnancy prolongation 6.6 wk.
Regenstein et al [49]	Observational case control	II-2	151	CPTL	No difference in the incidence of gestational diabetes or glucose intolerance between subcutaneous and oral groups
Allbert et al [73]	Observational cohort	II-2	64	RPTL	PPI was 0.86 and 0.72 for the pump and oral group, respectively.
Perry et al [84]	Descriptive case series	III	8709	CPTL	Continuous terbutaline infusion is associated with much fewer adverse effects than previously reported literature on intravenous terbutaline or ritodrine therapy suggest.
Elliott et al [97]	Retrospective cohort	II-2	21	CPTL 15 triplets 6 quadruplets	Estimated $18,150 savings per pregnancy. Only 2 (13%) of the 15 triplets and 1 (17%) of the 6 quadruplets delivered because of tocolytic failure. Mean GAD 33 wk for both groups.
Wenstrom et al [82]	Randomized control trial	I	42	CPTL	Three arm study: 15 terbutaline pump, 15 oral terbutaline, 12 saline pump. Significant methodologic flaw in that patients crossed over between groups while in study (patients on oral terbutaline or saline pump were switched to terbutaline pump if therapy failed). No electronic contraction monitoring or daily nursing contact. Tocolytic therapy was not individualized for each patient. Study underpowered in that it did not contain enough patients to show a difference between groups. No difference in outcomes between groups.
Guinn et al [83]	Randomized control trial	I	52	CPTL	Overall dropout rate 38%. Thirteen patients in the terbutaline group completed this study and 19 patients in the placebo group. Advanced median cervical dilatation of 3 cm, effacement of 50% at start. Tocolytic therapy was not individualized for each patient. No electronic contraction monitoring or daily nursing contact. Study was underpowered and showed no difference in outcomes between groups.
Lam et al [76]	Observational cohort	II-2	256	RPTL	Patients served as their own control. Subcutaneous terbutaline therapy prolonged pregnancy greater than oral terbutaline 4.4 ± 2.6 wk compared with 2.7 ± 2.2 wk.

(continued on next page)

Table 1 (continued)

Study	Research design	Quality of evidence	N	Population	Comments
Berkus et al [98]	Descriptive case series	III	7	CPTL	Low-dose, continuous subcutaneous terbutaline infusion had no effect on insulin sensitivity in nondiabetic patients, in contrast to oral terbutaline.
Hammersley et al [99]	Descriptive case series	III	70	RPTL 52 singletons 11 twins 7 triplets	Inclusion criterion: preterm labor or cervical shortening < 3 cm or 50% funneling. Mean cervical length 2.6 ± 0.9 cm at initiation of therapy. Seventy-six percent of desired pregnancy prolongation was achieved.
Lam et al [77]	Observational cohort	II-2	386	RPTL 386 twins	34 ± 19.8 versus 19.3 ± 15.3 days in utero gained with subcutaneous therapy compared with oral therapy.
Ambrose et al [100]	Observational case control	II-2	180	CPTL 76 twins	Outpatient-administered subcutaneous terbutaline shown to be a cost-effective and viable alternative vs inpatient-administered subcutaneous terbutaline.
Elliott et al [106]	Observational case control	II-2	144	144 quadruplets	Outpatient therapy cost $30,270 less per patient and is associated with a statistically significant better chance of delivery ≥ 32 wk than inpatient.
Elliott et al [80]	Observational cohort	II-2	104	RPTL 104 triplets	Mean pregnancy prolongation on pump 5.4 ± 3.4 wk versus 2.8 ± 2.2 wk for oral treatment.
Fleming et al	Observational case control	II-2	284	RPTL	37.3% of nifedipine patients delivered <35 wk compared with 19.7% of subcutaneous terbutaline patients. Subcutaneous terbutaline patients cost $6,945 less per pregnancy.
Lam et al [108]	Observational case control	II-2	706	RPTL 706 twins	Total maternal and nursery charges were $17,109 less for patients treated with subcutaneous terbutaline compared with oral treatment.
Elliott et al	Descriptive case series	III	9359	CPTL 7028 singletons 1946 twins 385 triplets	Extremely low incidence of serious adverse events. GAD was 36.6 wk in the singletons, 34.9 wk in the twins, and 32.8 wk in the triplets. Authors conclude therapy a viable and safe option for outpatient management.

Author	Study type	Evidence level	N	Group	Description
Hamersley et al [107]	Descriptive case series	III	6	Twins with delayed-interval delivery	The median pregnancy prolongation achieved following delivery of the first-born nonviable twin was 93 d.
Viscarello et al [109]	Observational case control	II-2	40	CPTL 40 triplets	Proactive dose acceleration protocol achieved significantly better outcomes than standard dosing.
Viscarello et al [101]	Observational case control	II-2	59	Higher order multiples 56 triplets 3 quadruplets	A comprehensive clinical pathway including subcutaneous terbutaline proved significantly better outcome (35.1 ± 1.6 versus 31.6 ± 3.1 wk GAD) compared with concurrent local standard of care. Of the 12 patients whose GAD was <32 wk, 1 received the comprehensive clinical pathway including subcutaneous terbutaline, compared with 11 who received the concurrent local standard of care.
Jones et al [102]	Descriptive case series	III	1691	RPTL	Over 57% of women experienced PTD within 1 week of DC of subcutaneous terbutaline. Early discontinuation of subcutaneous terbutaline places a pregnancy at risk for PTD.
Morrison et al	Observational case control	II-2	60	RPTL	Among patients with recurrent preterm labor, the use of subcutaneous terbutaline infusion significantly prolongs pregnancy while decreasing the likelihood of the rate of low birth weight (2500 g) infants, the need for admission to NICU, and duration of being hospitalized. For every dollar spent on subcutaneous terbutaline, there was a saving of $4.67 on the charges of newborns' stay in the hospital.
Lam et al [87]	Observational case control	II-2	558	RPTL	70.6% of subcutaneous therapy patients reached at least 36 wk compared with 56.6% of oral therapy patients. Subcutaneous therapy patients cost $5286 less.
Roman A et al [103]	Matched cohort	II-2	260	Twins in CPTL	>7 d prolongation of pregnancy in over 86% of cases.
Gaziano E et al [104]	Matched cohort	II-2	1079	CPTL	Outpatients obtained statistically better antepartum days, pregnancy prolongation, GAD, delivery <35 wk, and cost. Total average cost outpatient was $17,375 vs $39,040 inpatient.
Rebarber A et al [105]	Matched cohort	II-2	783	CPTL	86% of patients had their pregnancy prolonged >7 d.

Abbreviations: CPTL, current preterm labor (an initial episode of preterm labor stabilized and subcutaneous terbutaline infusion started); GAD, gestational age at delivery; PPI, pregnancy prolongation index; PTD, preterm delivery; RPTL, recurrent preterm labor (subcutaneous terbutaline infusion started at second occurrence of PTL after stabilization).

Safety

Perry and colleagues [84] found that subcutaneous terbutaline infusion for women with stabilized preterm labor is associated with much fewer adverse effects than previously reported β-agonist therapy. In a review of 8709 women receiving subcutaneous terbutaline infusion therapy for maintenance tocolysis, cardiac events including chest pain, EKG changes, arrhythmias, and cardiac arrest occurred with an incidence of 0.22%. Pulmonary edema developed in 0.32% of patients.

Elliott and colleagues [85] more recently reported on the incidence of subcutaneous pump therapy–related adverse side effects. A total of 9359 patients with singleton, twin, and triplet pregnancies were studied. Data were obtained from the national network of Matria Health Care patient service centers. Transient medication side effects were reported by 1447 (15.5%) patients. Severe adverse events were identified in 12 patients either during treatment with subcutaneous pump therapy (N = 4) or following discontinuation of therapy (N = 8). The most frequent, serious side effect was pulmonary edema (N = 9). There was no maternal mortality in this study, although mortality has been reported in women receiving subcutaneous pump therapy. In one case reported in 1992 [86] a patient pregnant with twins had been receiving subcutaneous pump therapy for 1 week before reporting severe chest pain and shortness of breath. The death was attributed to cardiac arrhythmia. Another woman died in the hospital from a ruptured iliac artery aneurysm during treatment with intravenous $MgSO_4$ after subcutaneous pump therapy was discontinued. In the report by Elliott and colleagues [85], the overall incidence of severe adverse events in women receiving subcutaneous pump therapy was low and the therapy was generally well tolerated. They recommended patients with comorbidity (ie, infection, preeclampsia, cardiac conditions) or concomitant tocolysis with intravenous $MgSO_4$ be closely assessed for development of serious events.

Costs

Lam and colleagues [87] also compared the clinical and cost effectiveness of using continuous subcutaneous terbutaline versus oral tocolytics following recurrent preterm labor. A total 558 women with singleton pregnancies were studied (279 per group). The oral group had less gestational gain following recurrent preterm labor than the subcutaneous pump therapy group (28.4 ± 19.8 days versus 33.9 ± 19 days, $P < .001$). The subcutaneous pump therapy group had less per patient charges for antepartum hospitalization ($3986 ± $6895 versus $5495 ± $7131, $P = .009$) and nursery ($7143 ± $20,048 versus $15,050 ± $32,648, $P < .001$). Outpatient charges were less for the oral group ($1390 ± $1152 versus $5520 ± $3292, $P < .001$). Overall costs for those in the subcutaneous pump therapy group were $5286 less per pregnancy compared with the oral group. In this population, continuous subcutaneous terbutaline infusion

Box 3. Essential components of the therapeutic program

1. Screen all patients for risk factors for preterm labor.
2. Establish baseline cervical status at the first prenatal visit.
3. Enroll at-risk patients in preterm labor education programs by 18 weeks' gestation.
4. Avoid prophylactic tocolysis with oral β-adrenergic agents, because this only leads to down-regulation of the β-receptors.
5. Advise bed rest and moderate hydration, if increased uterine activity is present.
6. Hospitalize and treat aggressively with parenteral tocolytics, if cervical change is documented. Do not wait for advanced cervical dilation (≥ 3 cm).
7. Rule out pathologic causes of preterm labor, such as infection, abruption, polyhydramnios, and congenital anomalies.
8. Use intravenous $MgSO_4$ as the primary tocolytic agent of choice, because it causes less maternal side effects and does not down-regulate the β-receptors, which may later be needed for long-term tocolysis.
9. Consider ambulatory tocolysis only after the patient has been stabilized on parental tocolytics.
10. Respect contraindications to tocolytic use.
11. Select a tocolytic agent to maximize efficacy and minimize toxicity on a patient-specific basis.
12. Titrate tocolytic dosage to end-organ effect (decrease of uterine activity) rather than toxicity (tachycardia or other side effects).
13. Monitor for signs of recurrent preterm labor.
14. Provide close nursing support.
15. Readmit patients with recurrent preterm labor for reinfusion with intravenous $MgSO_4$ tocolysis.
16. Use a sequential approach for tocolysis in recurrent preterm labor.
17. Allow a 24- to 48-hour intravenous $MgSO_4$ drug holiday in patients who experience a β-adrenergic tocolytic breakthrough.
18. Consider the terbutaline pump therapy for select patients: recurrent preterm labor; twins and higher-order multiples; intolerance of oral therapy; hospitalized patients stable on parenteral $MgSO_4$; advanced cervical change (stable); repeated episodes of breakthrough; and rehospitalization without advanced cervical change.

19. Use uterine activity monitoring to adjust bolus terbutaline therapy. Using the terbutaline pump without home uterine activity monitoring is like using an insulin pump without a glucometer.
20. Individualize tocolytic dosing. The patient's weight and volume of distribution should be carefully considered.

was both a clinically beneficial and cost-effective treatment following recurrent preterm labor.

It is estimated that subcutaneous pump therapy administered through the programmable pump in an ambulatory setting has been used in tens of thousands of pregnancies with excellent safety profiles and good outcome statistics [82,83]. Of the 39 reports in the world's literature, 37 demonstrate significant prolongation of the pregnancy compared with oral or no maintenance therapy. Pregnancy prolongation averaged 6.4 ± 2.8 weeks, which was double that of the control group, which only averaged 3.2 ± 6.6 weeks after treatment. These composite results (Table 1) support the authors' original findings [16,49,72–78, 80,82–84,87–110]. Most of these studies were in patients who were at very high risk for preterm delivery, with nine having populations of recurrent preterm labor and five involving multifetal gestations. Women with twin and higher-order multiple pregnancies at significant risk for preterm delivery constitute

Box 4. Contraindications to use of β-adrenergic agents

Relative contraindications

Advanced cervical dilation (>5 cm)
Maternal cardiac disease
Maternal pulmonary disease
Hyperthyroidism
Uncontrolled diabetes mellitus
Fetal anomaly
Fetal growth restriction

Absolute contraindications

Placental abruption
Eclampsia or severe preeclampsia
Heavy bleeding from any cause
Chorioamnionitis
Fetal death
Lethal fetal anomaly

a select group for whom this comprehensive model of management may be most appropriate.

Therapeutic principles for preterm labor treatment

The early diagnosis of preterm labor and immediate intervention is the essential component in halting the preterm labor process. Box 3 presents the essential components of the therapeutic program. This program is based on the authors' experience and that of other authors [6,67,111]. Box 4 lists contraindications to tocolytic use.

Summary

Of the numerous β-adrenergic medications used in the past 30 years, terbutaline was one of the first and remains the most enduring and popular. This widespread use can be attributed to physician confidence in terbutaline's efficacy, safety, and versatility in clinical practice. It is the only tocolytic agent that can be administered by the oral route; subcutaneously (intermittent and pump); and by intravenous infusion. Terbutaline is commonly used for acute and maintenance tocolysis. It is also the medication of choice for rescue tocolysis for uterine tetany in term labor and external cephalic version. Research efforts on subcutaneous pump therapy have been particularly active and interesting, yielding valuable new information on the roles of tachyphylaxis, LAHF, circadian patterns of preterm labor, sequential tocolysis, patient individualized therapy, and models for reducing cost of care. Current use of terbutaline involves lower-dose therapy (subcutaneous pump therapy) and sequential use of medications that do not bind to the β-adrenergic-receptor ($MgSO_4$, indomethacin, and nifedipine.) It is clear, however, that tocolytics alone are by no means a panacea for preventing preterm birth. Treatment success can be limited by adverse side effects. Proper monitoring and surveillance of patients on terbutaline tocolysis is warranted. Minor side effects are common; major side effects are rare and multifactorial. Particular attention should be given to patients with multifetal gestation, underlying infection, fluid overload, and cardiopulmonary disease. Since adoption of safety guidelines, the reported rates of adverse events have been dramatically decreased. The armamentarium has been severely limited. Established medications (ie, ritodrine) have been eliminated, and widely used medications (terbutaline, $MgSO_4$, and nifedipine) have not been granted regulatory approval. Newly formulated tocolytic agents will not be available because pharmaceutical companies do not want to bear the cost and risk of scale studies for the low usage rate [88,112–114]. The ultimate goal of achieving a term delivery with reduction in the incidence of low–birth weight infants will provide the greatest contribution in improving perinatal outcome in the future. Toward this goal, patients in preterm labor will often be willing to do anything to secure the health and well-being of their unborn children. It is the responsibility of physicians to ensure that their willingness to sacrifice remains within the realm of reason and safety.

References

[1] Caritis SN, Darby MJ, Chan L. Pharmacologic treatment of preterm labor. Clin Obstet Gynecol 1988;31:635–51.

[2] Lam F, Elliott J, Jones S, et al. Clinical issues surrounding the use of terbutaline sulphate for preterm labor. Obstet Gynecol Surv 1998;53:s85–95.

[3] Creasy RK, Katz M. Basic research and clinical experience with β-adrenergic tocolytics in the United States. In: Fuchs F, Stubblefield PG, editors. Preterm birth: causes prevention and management. Toronto: Macmillan; 1984. p. 150–70.

[4] Iams JD, Creasy RK. Preterm labor and delivery. In: Creasy RK, Resnick R, editors. Maternal - fetal medicine: principles and practice. 5th edition. Philadelphia: WB Saunders; 2004. p. 623–61.

[5] Simhan H, Caritis S. Inhibition of preterm labor. In: Rose BD, editor. Up-To-Date online. 2005;12:1–21.

[6] Lam F, Gill P. Subcutaneous terbutaline therapy in triplet gestation. In: Keith LG, Blickstein I, editors. Triplet pregnancies and their consequences. New York: Parthenon; 2002. p. 181–202.

[7] Nageotte MP. Prevention and treatment of preterm labor in twin gestation. Clin Obstet Gynecol 1990;33:61–8.

[8] Creasy RK. Preterm labor and delivery. In: Creasy RK, Resnick R, editors. Maternal-fetal medicine: principles and practice. Philadelphia: WB Saunders; 1984. p. 415–43.

[9] Alumbaugh KA. Off-label prescribing: practice management. Philadelphia (PA): American College of Obstetricians and Gynecologists; 1999.

[10] Berg G, Andersson RGG, Rygen G. β-Adrenergic receptors in human myometrium during pregnancy: changes in the number of receptors after β-mimetic treatment. Am J Obstet Gynecol 1985;151:392–6.

[11] Casper RF, Lye SJ. Myometrial desensitization to continuous but not to intermittent beta-adrenergic agonist infusion in sheep. Am J Obstet Gynecol 1986;154:301.

[12] Fredholm BB, Lunell N, Persson B, et al. Development of tolerance to the metabolic actions of β2-adrenoceptor stimulating drugs. Acta Obstet Gynecol Scand Suppl 1982;18:53–9.

[13] Mickey J, Tate R, Lefkowitz RJ. Subsensitivity of adenylate cyclase and decreased β-adrenergic receptor binding after chronic exposure to (-) isoproterenol in vitro. J Biol Chem 1975; 250:5727.

[14] Ryden G, Rolf G, Andersson G, et al. Is the relaxing effect of β-adrenergic agonists on the human myometrium only transitory? Acta Obstet Gynecol Scan Suppl 1982;108:47.

[15] Swillens S, Lefort E, Barber R, et al. Consequences of hormone-induced desensitization of adenylate cyclase in intact cells. Biochem J 1980;188:169.

[16] Lam F, Gill P, Smith M, et al. Use of the subcutaneous terbutaline pump for long-term tocolysis. Obstet Gynecol 1988;72:810–3.

[17] Newman RB, Gill PJ, Campion S. Antepartum ambulatory tocodynamometry: the significance of low-amplitude, high- frequency contractions. Obstet Gynecol 1987;70:701.

[18] Kawarabayashi T, Kuriyama K, Kishikawa T. Clinical features of small contraction wave recorded by an external tocodynamometer. Am J Obstet Gynecol 1988;158:474–8.

[19] Nakae S. Analysis of uterine contraction in late pregnancy and premature labor. Acta Obstet Gynaecol Jpn 1978;30:1637.

[20] Warkentin B. Die uterine aktivitat in der spatschwangerschaft. Z Geburtshilfe Perinat 1976; 180:225.

[21] Scheerer L, Katz MM. Home monitoring for preterm labor. In: Parer JT, editor. Antepartum and intrapartum management. Philadelphia: Lea and Febiger; 1989. p. 32–52.

[22] Newman RB, Gill PJ, Campion S, et al. The influence of fetal number on antepartum uterine activity. Obstet Gynecol 1989;73:695.

[23] Dahlberg NL. A perinatal center based antepartum homecare program. J Obstet Gynecol Neonatal Nurs 1988;17:30–4.

[24] Knuppel RA, Lake MF, Watson DL, et al. Preventing preterm birth in twin gestation: home uterine activity monitoring and perinatal nursing support. Obstet Gynecol 1990;76:24S–7S.

[25] Morrison JC, Chauhan SP, Carroll CS. Current status of home uterine activity monitoring. Clin Perinatol 2003;30:757–801.

[26] Katz M, Gill PJ, Newman RB. Detection of preterm labor by ambulatory monitoring of uterine activity: a preliminary report. Obstet Gynecol 1986;68:773–8.

[27] Katz M, Gill PJ, Newman RB. Detection of preterm labor by ambulatory monitoring of uterine activity for the management of oral tocolysis. Am J Obstet Gynecol 1986;154: 1253–6.

[28] Schwenzer TH, Schumann R, Halberstadt E. The importance of 24 hour cardiotocographic monitoring during tocolytic therapy. In: Jung H, Lamberti G, editors. Beta-mimetic drugs in obstetrics and perinatology. New York: Thieme-Stratton; 1982. p. 60.

[29] Zahn V. Uterine contractions during pregnancy. J Perinat Med 1984;12:107.

[30] Arakai R. The investigations of the effect of daily activity on the uterine contractions during pregnancy. Acta Obstet Gynecol Jpn 1984;36:589.

[31] Lam F. Miniature pump infusion of terbutaline: an option in preterm labor. Contemp Obstet Gynecol 1989;33:53.

[32] Newton ER. Antepartum care in multiple gestation. Semin Perinatol 1986;10:19–29.

[33] Marivate M, DeVilliers KQ, Fairbrother P. Effect of prophylactic outpatient administration of fenoterol on the time of onset of spontaneous labor and fetal growth rate in twin pregnancy. Am J Obstet Gynecol 1977;128:707.

[34] Skjaerris J, Aberg A. Prevention of prematurity in twin pregnancy by orally administered terbutaline. Acta Obstet Gynecol Scand 1982;108:39.

[35] Cetrulo CL, Freeman RK. Ritodrine HCL for the prevention of premature labor in twin pregnancies. Acta Genet Med Gemollol (Roma) 1976;25:321.

[36] O'Connor MC, Murphy H, Dalymple IJ. Double blind trial of ritodrine and placebo in twin pregnancy. Br J Obstet Gynaecol 1979;86:706.

[37] Goldberg RL. The management of preterm labor. Obstet Gynecol 2002;100:1020–37.

[38] Blickstein I. Maternal mortality. In: Blickstein I, Keith LG, editors. Multiple pregnancy: epidemiology, gestation and perinatal outcome. London: Taylor & Francis; 2005. p. 492–9.

[39] Streitman D, Caritis SN, Parilla BV. Should maintenance tocolytics play a role in the prevention of preterm birth? Contemp Obstet Gynecol 2001;46:11.

[40] How HY, Hughes SA, Vogel RL, et al. Oral terbutaline in the outpatient management of preterm labor. Am J Obstet Gynecol 1995;173:1518–22.

[41] Meirowitz NB, Anath CV, Smulian JC, et al. Value of maintenance therapy with oral tocolytics: a systematic review. J Matern Fetal Med 1999;8:177–83.

[42] Sanchez-Ramos L, Kaunitz AM, Gaudier FL, et al. Efficacy of maintenance therapy after acute tocolysis: a meta analysis. Am J Obstet Gynecol 1999;181:484–90.

[43] Canadian Preterm Labor Investigators Group. Treatment of preterm labor with the beta-adrenergic agonist ritodrine. N Engl J Med 1992;327:308.

[44] Beall M, Edgar B, Paul R, et al. A comparison of ritodrine, terbutaline, and magnesium sulfate for the suppression of preterm labor. Am J Obstet Gynecol 1985;153:857–9.

[45] Valenzuela G, Cline S. Use of magnesium sulphate in premature labor that fails to respond to β-mimetic drugs. Am J Obstet Gynecol 1982;143:718.

[46] Miller JM, Keane M, Horger EO. A comparison of magnesium sulphate and terbutaline for the arrest of premature labor: a preliminary report. J Reprod Med 1982;27:348–51.

[47] Hollander D, Nagey D, Pupkin M. Magnesium sulphate and ritodrine hydrochloride: a randomized comparison. Am J Obstet Gynecol 1987;156:631.

[48] Elliott JP. Magnesium sulfate as a tocolytic agent. Am J Obstet Gynecol 1983;147:277.

[49] Regenstein AC, Belluomini J, Katz M. Terbutaline tocolysis and glucose intolerance. Obstet Gynecol 1993;81:739–41.

[50] Weintraub Z, Solovechick M, Reichman B, et al. Effect of maternal tocolysis on the incidence of severe periventricular/intraventricular hemorrhage in very low birthweight infants. Arch Dis Child Fetal Neonatal Ed 2001;85:F13.

[51] Ozcan T, Turan C, Ekici E, et al. Ritodrine tocolysis and neonatal intraventricular-para-ventricular hemorrhage. Gynecol Obstet Invest 1995;39:60.

[52] Laros Jr RK, Kitterman JA, Heilbron D, et al. Outcome of very low birth weight infants exposed to beta-sympathomimetics in utero. Am J Obstet Gynecol 1991;164:1657.

[53] Palta M, Sadek M, Lim TS, et al. Association of tocolytic therapy with antenatal steroid administration and infant outcomes. Newborn Lung Project. Am J Perinatol 1998;15:87.

[54] Groome LJ, Goldenberg RL, Cliver SP, et al. Neonatal periventricular-intraventricular hemorrhage after maternal beta-sympathomimetic tocolysis. The March of Dimes Multicenter Study Group. Am J Obstet Gynecol 1992;167:873.

[55] Papatsonis DN, Kok JH, van Geijn HP, et al. Neonatal effects of nifedipine and ritodrine for preterm labor. Obstet Gynecol 2000;95:477.

[56] Hadders-Algra M, Touwen BCL, Huisjes HJ. Long-term follow-up of children prenatally exposed to ritodrine. Br J Obstet Gynaecol 1986;93:156.

[57] Rhodes MC, Seidler FJ, Abdel-Rahman A, et al. Terbutaline is a developmental neurotoxicant: effects on neuroproteins and morphology in cerebellum, hippocampus and somatosensory cortex. Am J Pharmacol Exp Ther 2004;308:529–37.

[58] Rhodes MC, Seidler FJ, Qiao D, et al. Does pharmacotherapy for preterm labor sensitize the developing brain to environmental neurotoxicants? Cellular and synaptic effects of sequential exposure to terbutaline and chlorpyrifos in neonatal rats. Toxicol Appl Pharmacol 2004;195: 203–17.

[59] Repke J, Niebyl J. The role of prostaglandin synthetase inhibitors in the treatment of preterm labor. Semin Reprod Endocrinol 1985;3:259.

[60] Niebyl JR, Witter FR. Neonatal outcome after indomethacin treatment for preterm labor. Am J Obstet Gynecol 1986;155:747–9.

[61] Vermillion ST, Scardo JA, Lashus AG, et al. The effect of indomethacin tocolysis on fetal ductus arteriosus constriction with advancing gestational age. Am J Obstet Gynecol 1997; 177:256.

[62] Dudley D, Hardie M. Fetal and neonatal effects of indomethacin used as a tocolytic agent. Am J Obstet Gynecol 1985;151:181–4.

[63] Wurtzel D. Prenatal administration of indomethacin as a tocolytic agent: effect on neonatal renal function. Obstet Gynecol 1990;76:689–92.

[64] Kirshon B, Moise KJ, Wasserstrum N, et al. Influence of short-term indomethacin therapy on fetal urine output. Obstet Gynecol 1988;72:51–3.

[65] Read MD, Wellby DE. The use of calcium antagonists (nifedipine) to suppress preterm labour. Br J Obstet Gynaecol 1986;93:933–7.

[66] Carr DB, Clark AL, Kernek K, et al. Maintenance oral nifedipine for preterm labor: a ran-domized clinical trial. Am J Obstet Gynecol 1999;181:822–7.

[67] Lam F, Gill P. Inhibition of preterm labor and subcutaneous terbutaline therapy. In: Blickstein I, Keith LG, editors. Multiple pregnancy: epidemiology, gestation and perinatal outcome. Lon-don: Taylor & Francis; 2005. p. 601–25.

[68] Gill P, Smith M, McGregor C. Terbutaline by pump to prevent recurrent preterm labor. Matern Child Nurs 1989;14:163–7.

[69] Sala DJ, Moise KJ. The treatment of preterm labor using a portable subcutaneous terbutaline pump. J Obstet Gynecol Neonatal Nurs 1989;19:108–15.

[70] Stanton RJ. Comanagement of the patient on subcutaneous terbutaline pump therapy. J Nurse Midwifery 1991;36:204–8.

[71] Garite TJ, Bentley DL, Hamer CA, et al. Uterine activity characteristics in multiple gestations. Obstet Gynecol 1990;76:56S–9S.

[72] Lam F, Gill PJ, Smith M, et al. Comparison of portable subcutaneous terbutaline pump and oral terbutaline treatment for long-term tocolysis: a randomized clinical trial. Presented at the Eight Annual Meeting, Society of Perinatal Obstetricians. Las Vegas, Nevada, February, 1988.

[73] Allbert JR, Johnson C, Roberts WE, et al. Tocolysis for recurrent preterm labor using a continuous subcutaneous infusion pump. J Reprod Med 1994;39:614.

[74] Allbert JR, Wise CA, Lou CH, et al. Subcutaneous tocolytic infusion therapy for patients at very high risk for preterm birth. J Perinatol 1992;12:28–31.

[75] Adkins RT, Van Hooydonk JE, Bressman PL, et al. Prevention of preterm birth: early detection and aggressive treatment with terbutaline. South Med J 1993;86:157–64.

[76] Lam F, Bergauer NK, Stanziano GJ, et al. Pregnancy prolongation and route of tocolytic administration in patients with singleton gestation. Am J Obstet Gynecol 1998;178:S180.

[77] Lam F, Bergauer NK, Coleman SK, et al. A comparison of gestational days gained with oral terbutaline vs. continuous subcutaneous terbutaline in women with twin gestations. J Perinatol 2000;20:408–13.

[78] Elliott JP, Radin TG. Quadruplet pregnancy: contemporary management and outcome. Obstet Gynecol 1992;80:421–4.

[79] Angel JL, Kalter CS, Morales WJ, et al. Aggressive perinatal care for high-order multiple gestations: does good perinatal outcome justify aggressive assisted reproductive techniques? Am J Obstet Gynecol 1999;181:253–9.

[80] Elliott JP, Bergauer NK, Jacques DL, et al. Pregnancy prolongation in triplet pregnancies: oral vs. continuous subcutaneous terbutaline. J Reprod Med 2001;46:975–82.

[81] Morrison JC, Chauhan SP, Carroll CS, et al. Continuous subcutaneous terbutaline administration prolongs pregnancy after recurrent preterm labor. Am J Obstet Gynecol 2003;188:1460–7.

[82] Wenstrom KD, Weiner CP, Merrill D, et al. A placebo-controlled randomized trial of the terbutaline pump for prevention of preterm delivery. J Perinatol 1997;14:87–91.

[83] Guinn DA, Goepfert AR, Owen J, et al. Terbutaline pump maintenance therapy for prevention of preterm delivery: a double-blind trial. Am J Obstet Gynecol 1998;179:874–8.

[84] Perry KG, Morrison JC, Rust OA. Incidence of adverse cardiopulmonary effects with low-dose continuous terbutaline infusion. Am J Obstet Gynecol 1995;173:1273–7.

[85] Elliott JP, Istwan NB, Rhea D, et al. The occurrence of adverse events in women receiving continuous subcutaneous terbutaline therapy. Am J Obstet Gynecol 2004;191:1277–82.

[86] Hudgens DR, Conradi SE. Sudden death associated with terbutaline sulphate administration. Am J Obstet Gynecol 1993;169:120–1.

[87] Lam F, Istwan NB, Jacques D, et al. Managing perinatal outcomes: the clinical- and cost-effectiveness of pharmacologic treatment of recurrent preterm labor. Manag Care 2003;12:39–46.

[88] Bisits A, Madsen G, Knox A, et al. The randomized Nitric Oxide Tocolysis Trial (RNOTT) for the treatment of preterm labor. Am J Obstet Gynecol 2004;191:683–90.

[89] Lam F, Graves WK, Peacock WG, et al. The impact of portable tocodynamometry and subcutaneous terbutaline pump therapy on preterm birth in a private obstetrical practice. Presented at the ACOG Districts VIII and IX Meeting. Las Vegas, Nevada, September 2, 1987.

[90] Gianopoulos J, Carlson N, Schumachen B. SQ terbutaline pump for premature labor. Am J Obstet Gynecol 1991;164:426.

[91] Jones P, Greenspan JS, Bochner CJ, et al. Continuous subcutaneous terbutaline infusion for the prevention of recurrent preterm labor. Am J Obstet Gynecol 1991;164:426.

[92] Fischer JR, Katz BL. Continuous subcutaneous infusion of terbutaline for suppression of preterm labor. Clin Pharm 1991;10:292–6.

[93] McGettigan MC, Bhutani VK, Rathbone A, et al. Prenatal β-mimetic exposure of the newborn: maternal oral vs. continuous infusion therapy. Pediatr Res 1991;30:62A.

[94] Lindenbaum C, Ludmir J, Teplick FB, et al. Maternal glucose intolerance and the subcutaneous terbutaline pump. Am J Obstet Gynecol 1992;166:925–8.

[95] Moise KJ, Sala DJ, Zurawin RK, et al. Continuous subcutaneous terbutaline pump therapy for premature labor, safety and efficacy. South Med J 1992;85:255–9.

[96] Weinbaum PJ, Olson M. The effect of subcutaneous infusion on uterine activity in patients at risk for preterm delivery. Am J Obstet Gynecol 1993;166:362.

[97] Elliott JP, Flynn MJ, Kaemmerer EL, et al. Terbutaline pump tocolysis in high order multiple gestation. J Reprod Med 1997;42:687–94.

[98] Berkus M, Langer O, Kigby K, et al. Effect of terbutaline pump on maternal glucose metabolism. Am J Obstet Gynecol 1999;180:S41.

[99] Hammersley S, Pinckert T, Gorman K, et al. The use of continuous subcutaneous terbutaline in a private maternal-fetal medicine practice. Obstet Gynecol 1999;93:67–8.

[100] Ambrose S, Jacques D, Stanziano G. Clinical and economic outcomes of continuous subcutaneous tocolysis. Obstet Gynecol 2001;97:47.

[101] Viscarello R, Griffith S, Charney L, et al. Outpatient management of higher order multiples with a comprehensive care plan improves outcome. Obstet Gynecol 2002;99:71.

[102] Jones JS, Istwan N. Pregnancy prolongation after discontinuation of subcutaneous tocolysis in singleton gestations. Obstet Gynecol 2003;101:4.

[103] Roman A, Rebarber A, Istwan N, et al. Clinical and demographic factors associated with spontaneous preterm delivery in twin pregnancies diagnosed with preterm labor at < 34 weeks. Am J Obstet Gynecol 2003;189:S123.

[104] Gaziano E, Wagner W, Rhea D, et al. Inpatient vs. outpatient surveillance for singleton pregnancies following inpatient treatment with magnesium sulfate for preterm labor. Presented at the Society for Gynecologic Investigation Annual Meeting. Houston, March 24–26, 2004.

[105] Rebarber A, Roman A, Istwan N. Factors associated with spontaneous preterm delivery in singleton gestations. Obstet Gynecol 2004;103(4).

[106] Elliott J, Istwan N, Jacques D, et al. Expectant management of the quadruplet pregnancy: inpatient or outpatient? Am J Obstet Gynecol 2001;185:110.

[107] Hamersley SL, Coleman SK, Bergauer NK, et al. Delayed –interval delivery in twin pregnancies. J Reprod Med 2002;47:125–30.

[108] Lam F, et al. Clinical and cost effectiveness of continuous subcutaneous terbutaline versus oral tocolytics for treatment of recurrent preterm labor in twin gestations. J Perinatol 2001;21: 444–50.

[109] Viscarello R, Griffith S, Jacques D, et al. The effect of proactive dose acceleration in triplets receiving continuous subcutaneous tocolysis. Obstet Gynecol 2002;99:12.

[110] Wolfsen R, Winn SK. Prolongation of twin pregnancy with magnesium sulphate / subcutaneous terbutaline pump therapy in the face of advanced cervical dilation and effacement. Am J Obstet Gynecol 1992;166:366.

[111] Rodts-Palenik S, Morrison JC. Tocolysis in triplet gestation. In: Keith LG, Blickstein I, editors. Triplet pregnancies and their consequences. New York: Parthenon; 2002. p. 149–73.

[112] Moutquin JM, Cabrol D, Fisk NM, et al. Effectiveness and safety of the oxytocin antagonist atosiban versus beta-adrenergic agonists in the treatment of preterm labour. Br J Obstet Gynaecol 2001;108:133–42.

[113] Moutquin JM, Sherman D, Cohen H, et al. Double-blind randomized controlled trial of atosiban and ritodrine in the treatment of preterm labor: a multicenter effectiveness and safety study. Am J Obstet Gynecol 2000;182:1191–9.

[114] Fleming A, Bonebrake R, Istwan N, et al. Pregnancy and economic outcomes in patients treated for recurrent preterm labor. J Perinatol 2004;4:223–7.

ELSEVIER
SAUNDERS

Obstet Gynecol Clin N Am
32 (2005) 485–500

OBSTETRICS AND
GYNECOLOGY
CLINICS
OF NORTH AMERICA

Magnesium Sulfate: The First-Line Tocolytic

David F. Lewis, MD

*Department of Obstetrics and Gynecology, Louisiana State University Health Sciences Center,
1501 Kings Highway, PO Box 33932, Shreveport, LA 71130–3932, USA*

Preterm labor and delivery continues to be the most common problem in obstetrics today and a major financial burden on the health care system. It has been estimated that this problem costs $15.5 billion (2002) in neonatal cost alone [1]. This estimate does not include the long-term medical conditions encountered by many preterm infants. Consequently, physicians are faced with the responsibility of identifying and implementing methods that can reduce the incidence of preterm delivery and the associated health care costs.

Over the last 50 years, extensive research has been conducted with the objective of preventing, predicting, and optimizing the outcome of patients with preterm labor. Despite these exhaustive efforts, the incidence of preterm birth has actually increased in recent years [2]. This unfavorable situation has had many obstetricians and researchers concluding that preterm labor is a syndrome with numerous etiologies that require unique treatment protocols [3]. A clear understanding of the fundamental causes coupled with optimal treatment protocols is needed to reduce the incidence of preterm labor and delivery.

Currently, the therapeutic foundation for treating preterm labor involves the use of tocolytics [4]. It is pertinent to point out that these drugs are used for arresting preterm labor regardless of the specific etiology contributing to the event. To date, the degree of success has been less than optimal despite the availability and use of several different tocolytic agents with different modes of action. The lack of successful treatment may well stem from the paucity of information about the initiating factors that ultimately lead to preterm labor. Labor results from a cascade of physiologic events. Consequently, to prevent preterm labor successfully, the therapeutic approach should be to focus on the

E-mail address: dlewi1@lsuhsc.edu

initial events of labor instead of attempting to inhibit the cascade of events culminating in preterm labor.

Of the various drugs used to arrest preterm labor, magnesium sulfate has emerged as the standard by which others are compared. This drug was first used by Steer and Petrie [5] as a tocolytic and later refined by Elliott [6]. In the United States, magnesium sulfate ranks as the tocolytic of choice by most obstetricians and perinatologists [7]. Knowledge about the pharmacology, mechanism of action, dosage, side effects, and the clinical efficacy of tocolytic agents should enable clinicians to provide better care for patients. Precise information about these factors, however, is often lacking.

Mechanism of action

Although magnesium sulfate has been used as a tocolytic since the early 1970s, information about its precise mechanism of action is still inadequate. Although the exact method is unknown, it is generally believed that the major action of magnesium sulfate relates to its inhibitory effect on calcium uptake and distribution. It seems that magnesium inhibits smooth muscle contractions by its direct effect on calcium activity. Magnesium modulates calcium uptake by reducing calcium binding and distribution in the myometrium [8]. Elevated magnesium levels inhibit calcium influx at cellular membranes by competing for calcium binding sites [9]. High titers of magnesium also increase the level of intracellular cyclic adenosine monophosphate and consequently reduce intracellular calcium [10]. Considerable in-depth research is needed to understand the mode of action of magnesium sulfate relative to preterm labor.

Pharmacology, dosage, and maternal complications

Serum levels between 5 and 8 ng/dL of magnesium are needed to attain myometrium inhibition [11,12]. Because of its rapid glomerular filtration, magnesium is excreted by the kidneys at a very high rate [13]: 75% of the drug is excreted during the initial infusion and over 90% is cleared within 24 hours [14]. Consequently, patients with abnormal renal function must be monitored carefully when magnesium sulfate is administered. Often, patients with renal impairment only require the initial loading dose to maintain an appropriate level for an extended time period. Although the optimal loading or starting doses are unknown, magnesium sulfate is usually administered intravenously with a loading dose of 4 to 6 g over a period of 15 to 30 minutes followed by a monitored dose of 2 to 6 g per hour [15]. The drug is then titrated to levels of 5 to 8 ng/dL or until adequate tocolysis is achieved. Some obstetricians contend that titration to clinical success is sufficient (Box 1) [16].

Box 1. Magnesium sulfate dosages

High: 6-g loading dose over 15–30 minutes followed by 2–6 g an hour.
Low: 4-g loading dose over 15–30 minutes followed by 2 g an hour.

Whether magnesium levels are checked every 4 to 6 hours or clinical effectiveness is used as an end point, patients must be evaluated for evidence of drug toxicity. Recognizing that, even though magnesium sulfate is the first-line agent, several areas of concern exist because of its few serious adverse side effects. Decreased or absent deep tendon reflexes represents an initial sign of toxicity. This condition can be evaluated readily by a trained nurse and is usually noted when the magnesium level exceeds 10 ng/dL. It is important to note that respiratory depression has been reported when levels greater than 15 ng/dL have been used. Myocardial depression has also been described at very high doses. Most patients who receive magnesium sulfate exhibit minor adverse side effects, such as a perception of being hot, flushy, and nauseous; vomiting; blurred or double vision; and lethargy. These side effects usually become more tolerable as the duration of drug exposure increases. Although rare, more serious side effects, such as hypothermia [17,18], osteoporosis [19], rhabdomyolysis [20], and kidney stones [21], have been described, magnesium sulfate is well tolerated and carries only a fraction of the side effects found with the β-mimetics [12,22]. For those patients who exhibit toxicity to magnesium sulfate, 1 g of calcium gluconate can be administered intravenously to reverse the side effects.

Contraindications to magnesium sulfate are uncommon. Myasthenia gravis is an absolute contraindication, however, because these patients experience respiratory arrest and require prolonged ventilator support when given magnesium sulfate. Additional contraindications include cardiac disease; renal impairment; and the concomitant use of a calcium channel blocker, which can cause profound hypotension [23].

Although serious complications associated with magnesium sulfate therapy are rare, they may be noted following errors in drug administration that occur when an inadvertent large bolus of the drug is administered. It is imperative that fluid balance be assessed during the period of drug administration because the rate of pulmonary edema following magnesium sulfate therapy has been reported as between 0% and 2% of cases [6]. The higher rates of pulmonary edema were noted in conjunction with tocolytic therapy for multifetal pregnancies, the use of several tocolytic agents, or their prolonged usage [24]. Although the etiology of pulmonary edema is uncertain, its occurrence is associated with occult infections, fluid imbalance, increased pulmonary permeability, and changes in osmotic pressure. The complications of pulmonary edema can be readily treated with

Table 1
Reported maternal and fetal side effects following magnesium sulfate therapy

Maternal

Short term	Long term	Toxicity
Lethargy	Osteoporosis	Absent deep tendon reflexes
Nausea	Tetany	Respiratory depression
Vomiting	Paralytic ileus	Cardiac arrhythmia
Flushed	Pulmonary edema	Cardiac arrest
Hot feeling	Hypothermia	Death
Headaches	Renal stones	
Constipation	Rhabdomyolysis	
Dry mouth		
Hypocalcemia		

Fetal

Short term	Long term
Decreased fetal movement	Decalcification of bones
Absent fetal breathing	
Decreased short-term variability of fetal heart	
Altered uterine blood flow	
Blunted fetal response	

Neonatal

Short term	High doses	Low doses
Hypermagnesemia	Neonatal death?	Neuroprotective
Hypocalcemia		
Lethargy		
Depressed Apgars		
Hypotonia		
Decalcification of bones		

furosemide. Even though magnesium sulfate is generally considered a relatively safe drug, it must be monitored closely throughout its administration, as is the case with all drugs (Table 1).

Fetal and neonatal effects

Magnesium sulfate also has several effects on the fetus and neonate. The drug rapidly reaches a steady state between maternal and fetal components because it readily crosses the placenta [13]. Although maternal and fetal serum and amniotic fluid levels appear linearly correlated, prolonged therapy can lead to higher levels in the fetus, which directly affects fetal urine output [25]. The primary neonatal side effects of magnesium sulfate tocolysis are lethargy, hypotonicity, and low Apgar scores [26]. These conditions are usually self-limiting and are resolved as the drug is systematically cleared after delivery. Antenatal side effects reported include decreased variability of the fetal heart rate [27,28], altered cerebral blood flow, and a depressed biophysical profile [27]. It should be noted that some authors found no change in the biophysical profile with magnesium sulfate tocolysis [29]. Additionally, prolonged usage (weeks or months) of magnesium sulfate has been associated with demineralization of fetal bone [30–32].

Several recent studies have suggested that magnesium sulfate may have a favorable neuroprotective effect on the neonate by lowering the incidence of cerebral palsy [33–35]. intraventricular hemorrhage, and mortality [36–38]. A prospective trial involving over 1000 preterm deliveries (before 30 weeks of gestation) included patients exposed to either low-dose magnesium sulfate or saline [39]. The results indicated that the frequencies of both cerebral palsy and motor delay were lower in the magnesium sulfate group than in those patients who received saline. Because this trial used a magnesium sulfate dosage lower than that normally used for tocolysis, the data cannot be reasonably extrapolated to different protocols. These promising results, however, do confirm previously published data [33,34,37,38]. Even though several studies have suggested that high dosages of magnesium sulfate are associated with elevated neonatal death rates [40,41], other reports have not confirmed this finding [38,42]. The reports of several adverse fetal effects of magnesium sulfate should be compared with the possible outcomes of not using magnesium sulfate. Without this drug, a rapid preterm delivery might occur, which prevents full-dose corticosteroid therapy and results in higher neonatal morbidity and mortality (see Table 1).

General clinical efficacy

Magnesium sulfate was introduced as an obstetric tocolytic agent by Steer and Petrie [5]. In this classic study, patients were randomly assigned to receive magnesium sulfate, ethanol, or a dextrose solution placebo. The data showed that magnesium sulfate therapy arrested contractions for 24 hours in 77% of the patients receiving magnesium sulfate compared with 45% and 44% in the ethanol and dextrose groups, respectively. A subsequent statistical analysis of these data showed that the proportion of patients in the magnesium sulfate group had a significantly ($P<.01$) higher incidence of arrested contractions compared with the other two groups. Although these preliminary data laid the groundwork for the use of magnesium sulfate as a tocolytic, the outcome of the study by Steer and Petrie [5] was compromised by the use of a relatively low dosage of magnesium sulfate (4-g loading dose and 2 g per hour). Another descriptive study [43] involved 85 patients who received magnesium sulfate and 107 patients who received magnesium sulfate and oral isoxsuprine hydrochloride or terbutaline. In this report, 119 patients had intact membranes, whereas 73 had ruptured membranes. Successful tocolysis (delayed delivery by 48 hours) was achieved in 70.6% of patients with intact membranes and in 60.2% of patients with ruptured membranes. The authors concluded that magnesium sulfate was an effective tocolytic with minimal side effects, although pointing out that its efficacy in patients with ruptured membranes was controversial.

A retrospective study used data from 355 patients who received magnesium sulfate as a tocolytic agent, and 274 patients (77.2%) had intact membranes with cervical dilation ranging from 0 to more than 6 cm [6]. Delivery was delayed for over 48 hours in 208 (76%) of these 274 patients. This incidence is similar to the success rate of 77% found in a similar group of patients reported by Steer and Petrie [5]. Recognizing that the study by Elliott [6] in 1983 included different classifications of patients, such as singletons, twins, and those with intact or ruptured membranes, it nevertheless set the stage for widespread acceptance of magnesium sulfate as a tocolytic in the United States. Although a 1985 national survey by Taslimi et al [44] revealed that over 70% of practicing obstetricians and perinatologists used ritodrine as their primary tocolytic agent following the results from these three trials, the use of ritodrine rapidly decreased over the next decade (1980s) and magnesium sulfate became the primary tocolytic agent.

Magnesium sulfate versus placebo

Three studies comparing magnesium sulfate with placebo have been reported in the literature. Steer and Petrie [5] compared the data from 31 patients who received magnesium sulfate with 9 patients who received placebo. They found that uterine quiescence for 24 hours was attained in 77% of those patients who received magnesium sulfate versus 44% in the placebo group. Recognizing the small number of control patients, an ad hoc analysis of their data did show a statistically significant ($P<.1$) trend. These findings, however, seem compromised because of the relatively low dosages of magnesium sulfate administered (4-g loading dose followed by 2 g per hour maintenance dose). Cotton et al [45] studied 69 patients between 26 and 34 weeks of gestation with intact or ruptured membranes and used the same dose of magnesium sulfate as reported by Steer and Petrie [5]. The patients were randomized to magnesium sulfate, terbutaline, or placebo (5% dextrose in lactated Ringer's solution) groups. The delays to delivery times were similar between the 16 patients who received magnesium sulfate and the 19 who received placebo. Another study [46] involved 156 patients with intact membranes between 24 and 34 weeks of gestation. Patients were randomly assigned to receive either magnesium sulfate or normal saline. The time duration to delivery was similar between the groups (26.6 days for magnesium sulfate group and 22.4 days for placebo group).

Several points should be made about these three trials. First, the loading dose of magnesium sulfate was only 4 g, which is lower than that recommended by many clinicians. Second, excluding the study by Cox et al [46], which did allow the drug dosage to be increased by 1 g an hour (maximum 3 g an hour) after 1 hour if contractions persisted, all patients were maintained on 2 g magnesium sulfate per hour after the loading dose was administered. Third, the study by Cotton et al [45] seems confounded because the data from women with intact membranes were combined with the data from patients with ruptured membranes. Fourth, a power analysis was not performed before data collection to determine the number of patients needed to achieve statistically significant differences. Fifth, the sample size was small with a combined number of patients in these three studies representing 123 patients who received magnesium sulfate and 118 who received a placebo. The results from these three studies influenced the Cochrane database analysis by Crowther et al [47] to conclude that "no benefit was seen for magnesium sulfate." Nevertheless, the results from these three studies represent the only reported placebo-controlled trials and further emphasize the need for further research involving a large multicenter randomized trial.

Magnesium sulfate versus prostaglandin synthetase inhibitors

Many prospective randomized trials and retrospective analyses of data have been conducted to compare the efficacy of magnesium sulfate with other tocolytic agents, such as prostaglandin synthetase inhibitors, calcium channel blockers, nitroglycerin, β-mimetics, and various tocolytic combinations. Zuckerman et al [48] first introduced indomethacin as a tocolytic in 1974. Morales and Madhav [49] compared the effectiveness of magnesium sulfate relative to indomethacin by randomly assigning 52 patients to the magnesium sulfate group and 49 to an indomethacin group. Each patient had intact membranes and was less than 32 weeks of gestation. The results showed that the proportion of deliveries occurring more than 48 hours after initiating treatment was 85% and 90% in the magnesium sulfate and indomethacin groups, respectively. Also, the mean duration of prolonging delivery was similar between the two groups: 22.7 days for the magnesium sulfate group and 22.9 days for the indomethacin group. The only advantage noted for indomethacin was a decrease in the incidence (15% for magnesium sulfate and 0% for indomethacin) of adverse maternal side effects that required discontinuation of the drug.

Schorr et al [50] performed a prospective randomized trial on patients less than 32 weeks with intact membranes who received either intravenous magnesium sulfate or intramuscular ketorolac. The only difference noted was that the time period required to obtain uterine quiescence was significantly ($P<.05$) shorter in the ketorolac group (2.7 versus 6.2 hours). Adverse effects were not noted and discontinuation of neither drug was needed. Recently, McWhorter et al [51] compared the tocolytic efficacy of magnesium sulfate with rofecoxib (cyclo-oxygenase-2 inhibitor). They studied 214 patients between 22 and 34 weeks of gestation with intact membranes and found that delivery was similarly delayed for 48 hours in 90.4% and 88% of the pregnancies treated with rofecoxib and magnesium sulfate, respectively. A higher incidence of adverse side effects was found, however, in the magnesium sulfate group.

Magnesium sulfate versus calcium channel blockers

Results were found from two trials that compared magnesium sulfate with calcium channel blockers. Glock and Morales [52] reported that the effects of magnesium sulfate and oral nifedipine were similar in their ability to prevent delivery for over 48 hours. The use of either tocolytic agent resulted in a success rate exceeding 90%. Once patients successfully achieved tocolysis, the magnesium sulfate patients were given oral terbutaline, whereas the nifedipine patients had that medication continued. Four patients in the magnesium sulfate group required discontinuation of the drug because of adverse side effects. Another study by Larmon et al [53] compared intravenous magnesium sulfate with oral nicardipine. The only difference noted was that uterine quiescence was significantly ($P<.01$) more rapid in the 57 patients randomized to nicardipine (3.3 hours) than in the 65 patients treated with magnesium sulfate (5.3 hours). Similar to the report by Glock and Morales [52], adverse side effects were more prevalent in the magnesium sulfate–treated patients. The times to delivery were similar and no other differences were noted.

Magnesium sulfate versus nitroglycerin

Results from only one prospective randomized trial involving relatively few patients were found. El-Sayed et al [54] reported that magnesium sulfate was statistically ($P<.05$) more successful at arresting preterm labor (78.6% versus 37.5%) than was intravenous nitroglycerin. Although a higher proportion (25%) of patients who received nitroglycerin developed hypotension, the overall incidence of relatively minor adverse side effects was higher in the magnesium sulfate group. Only one patient in each group required the therapy to be discontinued.

Magnesium sulfate versus β-mimetics

A relatively large amount of comparative data exists for these two types of tocolytics. When magnesium sulfate was first introduced as a tocolytic agent, ritodrine was the most commonly used tocolytic agent and the only drug approved by the United States Food and Drug Administration for arresting preterm labor. Two separate studies [45,55] compared intravenous terbutaline with low-dose intravenous magnesium sulfate (4 g loading dose and 2 g per hour). Each study reported similar outcomes between the two groups. Conversely, a prospective study by Chau et al [56] randomly allocated 98 patients to either one of four groups: (1) subcutaneous terbutaline, (2) oral terbutaline, (3) intravenous magnesium sulfate, or (4) oral magnesium sulfate. They found no differences in the number of patients who delivered in less than 48 hours between the magnesium sulfate and terbutaline groups (10.9% and 21.2%, respectively). Additionally, the magnesium sulfate groups had a significantly higher ($P < .05$) proportion of term deliveries (≥ 37 weeks of gestation) than did the patients who received terbutaline (73.9% and 51.9%, respectively).

When Wilkins et al [57] compared the efficacy of ritodrine with magnesium sulfate in a prospective randomized trial comprising 120 patients in preterm labor, both drugs were found to provide excellent results in preventing preterm delivery for greater than 48 hours (96.3% for ritodrine and 92.3% for magnesium sulfate). More serious side effects were found, however, in the ritodrine group. The protocol called for adding the other drug if the first tocolytic was unsuccessful; additional drug therapy was required in 13 cases. The combination therapy resulted in 77% of patients experiencing side effects and was deemed not beneficial over single-agent therapy. A 1985 study designed to evaluate secondary treatment for initial tocolytic drug failures randomized 176 patients to intravenous magnesium sulfate, ritodrine, or terbutaline [58]. The authors concluded that each of these three drugs produced similar effects, although intravenous administration of terbutaline had considerably more unfavorable side effects. When evaluating the results from studies comparing the merits of magnesium sulfate and intravenous β-mimetics for delaying labor for periods greater than 48 hours, the conclusion is reached that there was not a clinically significant difference between the two drugs. Although patients who received magnesium sulfate had more side effects, those side effects were less serious than in the patients who received intravenous ritodrine or intravenous terbutaline.

Combination tocolytic therapy

Several investigators have evaluated the effectiveness of magnesium sulfate in combination with another drug. When Hatjis [59] treated 65 idiopathic preterm labor patients with ritodrine, 30 patients were unresponsive. Those 30 patients were then given intravenous magnesium sulfate with successful tocolysis in 18 (60%) of the initially unresponsive patients. The authors concluded that magnesium sulfate may improve pregnancy outcome in patients who did not initially respond to ritodrine treatment. Later, Hatjis et al [60] randomly assigned preterm labor patients to a ritodrine group and others to a cohort that received both ritodrine and magnesium sulfate. The authors concluded that combination therapy was superior based on the finding that those patients receiving combination therapy had a significantly ($P < .05$) higher success rate (59% versus 34% $P < .05$) than those who only received ritodrine.

Ogburn et al [61] studied the outcome of 23 patients who were initially unresponsive to single-agent tocolysis when subsequently given magnesium sulfate and ritodrine or terbutaline. Although 61% (14 of 23) of the patients who received combination therapy delayed delivery for 48 hours or more, 22% (5 of 23) developed pulmonary edema. Coleman [62] found that 95 preterm labor patients managed with magnesium sulfate and ritodrine had a complication rate of 21%, which necessitated cessation of tocolysis. Nevertheless, the author concluded that combination therapy was efficacious. Kosasa et al [63] reported the results from 1000 patients who were treated with combination intravenous magnesium sulfate and terbutaline. The patients were treated with both drugs continuously from the diagnosis of preterm labor until delivery. The 751 patients with intact membranes had an average delay in delivery of 61 days, whereas the 249 patients with ruptured membranes delayed delivery by 21 days. Complications of the therapy were noted in 56% of patients with intact membranes and in 41% of patients with ruptured membranes.

Lewis et al [64] compared the efficacy of magnesium sulfate alone with the combination of magnesium sulfate and indomethacin in patients who had idiopathic preterm labor with advanced cervical dilation (3 cm or greater). The 21 patients treated with combination therapy had a significantly ($P < .001$) longer average delay in delivery (15.4 versus 2.9 days $P < .001$). Adverse side effects were not found in either group. The authors concluded that combination tocolysis with magnesium sulfate and indomethacin seemed to be safe and effective in patients with advanced cervical dilation.

Clinical efficacy

Although several of the studies reported similarities in the duration of pregnancy when a magnesium sulfate treatment group was compared with a placebo control group, the obvious question arises, "Why has this drug become the first line of therapy for idiopathic preterm labor"? To address this question, examination of the experimental design used in these reports is necessary. All of the patients in these trials were initially loaded with only 4 g of magnesium sulfate, and most were maintained on 2 g for 1 hour. Even though Cox et al [46] allowed the dosage of magnesium sulfate to be increased to 3 g per hour, none of the published studies showed that the drug was titrated until a successful cessation of uterine contraction was evident. Such titration of drugs is currently the common practice among obstetricians. Nevertheless, the results from the literature lead one to conclude that achieving adequate tocolysis with magnesium sulfate is questionable [47].

To evaluate the tocolytic effectiveness of magnesium sulfate judiciously, however, the published results in which the tocolytic effects of nonsteroidal compounds are compared with those of magnesium sulfate should also be considered. Several comprehensive evaluations have concluded that nonsteroidal compounds are the only drugs documented to inhibit preterm labor. The results from three prospective randomized trials [49,51,52] have shown, however, that the tocolytic response from nonsteroidal compounds is as efficacious as that found with magnesium sulfate. It should be noted that the treatment protocol used in each of these three trials called for aggressive tocolysis (6-g loading dose of magnesium sulfate and maintenance doses of 2 g up to 6 g per hour) to achieve favorable labor quiescence. Adherence to the adequate loading and maintenance magnesium sulfate dosages and the duration of treatment seem necessary for successful tocolytic outcomes. A successful delay in delivery was achieved in over 85% of the studies using higher dosages of magnesium sulfate as compared with considerably lower success rates when decreased dosages of magnesium sulfate were used.

The clinical data have shown that low-dose magnesium sulfate is not very effective at preventing preterm delivery. Aggressive magnesium sulfate therapy has a success rate of 85% or greater at 48 hours, however, which then allows sufficient time for administering corticosteroids. A cautionary note is that combining magnesium sulfate with other tocolytics markedly increases maternal side effects and must be done cautiously.

An analysis was performed of the clinical trials available (Table 2). The trials were broken into three groups based on the dosage of magnesium sulfate used: (1) low-dose magnesium sulfate (4-g loading dose and 2 g an hour constant infusion); (2) medium-dose magnesium sulfate (4-g loading dose and >2 g an hour constant infusion); or (3) high-dose magnesium sulfate (6-g loading dose and >2 g an hour constant infusion. Evaluating the trials in this manner revealed 174 patients received low-dose treatment, 462 patients received medium-dose

Table 2
Dosage of magnesium sulfate and success of tocolysis at 48 hours

Low dose (4-g load and 2 g an hour)

	No.	% success
Spisso et al [43]	119	64
Cotton et al [45]	10	70.6
Miller et al [55]	14	60
Steer and Petrie [5]	31	77.0
	174	70.7[a]

Medium dose (4-g load and ≥2 g an hour)

	No.	% success
Chau et al [56]	46	95.7
Wilkins et al [57]	66	92.3
Cox et al [46]	76	70
Elliott [6]	274	76
	462	79.2[a]

High dose (6-g load and ≥2 g an hour)

	No.	% success
Morales and Madhav [49]	52	85
Schorr et al [50]	43	84
McWhorter et al [51]	109	88
Glock and Morales [52]	41	93
Larmon et al [53]	65	94
	310	88.7[a]

[a] The differences in the proportion of successful outcomes among the three dosage groups were statistically significant (P <.01, chi-square).

treatment, and 310 patients received high-dose treatment. Success was defined as the ability to prevent delivery for 48 hours. Success rates improved as the dosage of magnesium sulfate increased (70.7% low-dose, 79.2% medium-dose, and 88.7% high-dose magnesium sulfate). This information suggests that high dosages of magnesium sulfate should become the standard if the goal is the prevention of preterm delivery for at least 48 hours.

Terrone et al [65] randomized patients after they received a loading dose of 4 g of magnesium sulfate. The patients then received either 2 g an hour constant infusion (low dose) or 5 g an hour constant infusion. The dosage was then adjusted by 1-g increments an hour to achieve tocolysis. The higher infusion rate took less time to achieve uterine quiescence and had a lower rate of treatment failures. These data suggest that aggressive management is important for achieving successful tocolysis.

Special clinical situations

Several clinical situations require consideration. Do cervical alterations after initiation of magnesium sulfate influence the prognosis? Data by Lewis et al [66] addressed this question. They assigned 126 patients to one of three groups: (1) those whose cervix changed after initiation of tocolysis (24 patients); (2) those whose cervix regressed (44 patients); and (3) those whose cervix remained unchanged (58 patients). Patients who had cervical progression after starting tocolysis had a shorter delay to delivery, delivered at an earlier gestational age, and were less likely to progress to term than the other two groups. Patients with cervical progression represent a group whose short-term goal includes the administration of corticosteroids.

Another question resides around the benefits of oral magnesium after successful intravenous magnesium sulfate tocolysis. Preliminary work by Martin et al [67] seems promising. These investigators also performed a prospective trial in which 54 patients were randomized to either 1 g of orally administered magnesium gluconate every 6 hours or to a placebo group [68]. No difference in the rate of preterm delivery was noted between the two groups and suggested, as do other data involving oral terbutaline, that oral magnesium gluconate does not prolong pregnancy in a high-risk group.

Should tocolysis be attempted after ruptured membranes? Results [69,70] demonstrated that high maternal complication rates may ensue and little benefit may occur if such a protocol was attempted. Conversely, more recent data indicate that tocolytic therapy following ruptured membranes seems beneficial [71,72]. The use of antibiotics in treating preterm premature rupture of the membranes has been found to prolong pregnancy. Presently, a large prospective trial is needed to determine the benefit of this therapy. Until such data are obtained, no standard can be reasonably established: some authorities advocate its use, whereas others find no benefit [70].

Is long-term therapy (treatment from diagnosis of preterm labor to delivery) more beneficial than short-term acute tocolysis? Several trials have described the results obtained from long-term use of intravenous magnesium sulfate [63,73,74]. One study compared the tocolytic effects of short- versus long-term therapies [73] and reported fewer neonatal complications following long-term treatment. Widespread acceptance of long-term therapy has not occurred, however, and several neonatal side effects have been ascribed to its use [75]. Currently, it seems that prospective trials are needed to obtain data in which long- and sort-term therapy protocols are compared.

Is weaning the drug necessary? A common medical practice is to slowly discontinue magnesium sulfate instead of abruptly stopping the drug. Lewis et al [76] completed a prospective randomized study to address this important question. A total of 141 patients were randomized to either slowly discontinuing magnesium sulfate therapy (72 patients) or abruptly stopping the drug (69 patients). The group whose treatment was gradually discontinued had a higher incidence of retocolysis with no apparent benefit in outcome. These results were probably influenced by the rapid clearance of the drug by the kidneys, which were no doubt responsible for the physiologic weaning. Consequently, the practice of weaning the drug does not seem to be beneficial.

Summary

Magnesium sulfate has become the first-line tocolytic for short-term use to arrest idiopathic preterm labor. The reasons for its acceptance include familiarity of the drug, ease of use, and the virtual absence of serious maternal and fetal side effects. Sufficient data exist showing its efficacy if used in higher doses (6-g load and 2–6 g per hour to achieve uterine quiescence). These findings place magnesium sulfate in the same category as other drugs, such as nonsteroidals, where success rates greater than 85% are common.

Side effects occur with any drug including magnesium sulfate. Most of the unfavorable maternal side effects are relatively mild and rarely require discontinuation of the drug. It is imperative to monitor patients who are given magnesium sulfate to prevent serious complications. Several benefits are associated with magnesium sulfate therapy including the ability to administer corticosteroids, the prolongation of pregnancy, and possibly preventing long-term neurologic sequelae in the newborn. It seems ironic that a drug used this frequently has not been studied more thoroughly. Currently, very few clinical research trials are being undertaken and the most efficacious use and success rate of magnesium sulfate remain unknown. Attention to treating preterm labor has shifted to seeking answers about the fundamental causes. Gathering information about the specific causes and designing tailor-made treatment protocols for each of the numerous potential causes seems essential. To accomplish this, scientifically sound research is needed to obtain answers about the important clinical questions surrounding magnesium sulfate.

References

[1] National Center for Health Statistics, Perinatal Overview. Available at: http://www.marchofdimes. com/peristats. Accessed May 16, 2005.
[2] Martin JA, Hamilton BE, Ventura SJ, et al. Births: final data for 2000. Natl Vital Stat Rep 2002; 50:1–101.
[3] Romero R, Mazor M, Munoz H, et al. The preterm labor syndrome. Ann N Y Acad Sci 1994; 734:414–29.
[4] Goldenberg RL. The management of preterm labor. Obstet Gynecol 2002;100:1020–37.
[5] Steer CM, Petrie RH. A comparison of magnesium sulfate and alcohol for the prevention of premature labor. Am J Obstet Gynecol 1977;129:1–4.
[6] Elliott JP. Magnesium sulfate as a tocolytic agent. Am J Obstet Gynecol 1983;147:277–84.
[7] Gordon MC, Iams JD. Magnesium sulfate. Clin Obstet Gynecol 1995;38:706–12.
[8] James MFM. Magnesium in obstetric anesthesia. Inter J Obstet Anes 1998;7:115.
[9] Ohki S, Ikura M, Zhang M. Identification of magnesium binding sites and the role of magnesium on target recognition by calmodulin. Biochemistry 1997;36:4309–16.
[10] Caritis SN, Darby MJ, Chan L. Pharmacologic treatment of preterm labor. Clin Obstet Gynecol 1988;31:635–51.
[11] Elliott JP. Magnesium sulfate as a tocolytic agent. Contemp Ob Gyn 1985;147:277–84.
[12] Hollander DI, Nagey DA, Pupkin MJ. Magnesium sulfate and ritodrine hydrochloride: a randomized comparison. Am J Obstet Gynecol 1987;156:631.
[13] Idama TO, Lindow SW. Magnesium sulphate: a review of clinical pharmacology applied to obstetrics. Br J Obstet Gynaecol 1998;105:260–8.
[14] Cruikshank DP, Pitkin RM, Donnelly E, et al. Urinary magnesium, calcium, and phosphate excretion during magnesium sulfate infusion. Obstet Gynecol 1981;58:430–4.
[15] Rodts-Palenik S, Morrison JC. Tocolysis: an update for the practitioner. Obstet Gynecol Surv 2002;57:S9–34.
[16] Madden C, Owen J, Hauth JC. Magnesium tocolysis: serum levels versus success. Am J Obstet Gynecol 1990;162:1177–80.
[17] Parsons MT, Owens CA, Spellacy WN. Thermic effects of tocolytic agents: decreased temperature with magnesium sulfate. Obstet Gynecol 1977;69:88–90.
[18] Rodis JF, Vintzileos AM, Campbell WA, et al. Maternal hypothermia: an unusual complication of magnesium sulfate therapy. Am J Obstet Gynecol 1987;156:435–6.
[19] Levav AL, Chan L, Wapner RJ. Long-term magnesium sulfate tocolysis and maternal osteoporosis in a triplet pregnancy: a case report. Am J Perinatol 1998;15:43–6.
[20] Matsuda Y, Nagayoshi Y, Kirihara N. Rhabdomyolysis during prolonged intravenous tocolytic therapy. J Perinat Med 2002;30:514–6.
[21] Sameshima H, Higo T, Kodama Y, et al. Magnesium tocolysis as the cause of urinary calculus during pregnancy. J Matern Fetal Neonatal Med 1997;6:296–7.
[22] Chau AC, Gabert HA, Miller JM. A prospective comparison of terbutaline and magnesium for tocolysis. Obstet Gynecol 1992;80:847.
[23] Anthony J, Johanson RG, Duley L. Role of magnesium sulfate in seizure prevention in patients with eclampsia and preeclampsia. Drug Saf 1996;15:188.
[24] Ramsey PS, Rouse DJ. Magnesium sulfate as a tocolytic agent. Semin Perinatol 2001;25:236–47.
[25] Hankins GDV, Hammond TL, Yeomans ER. Amniotic cavity accumulation of magnesium with prolonged magnesium sulfate tocolysis. J Reprod Med 1991;36:446–9.
[26] Petrie RH. Tocolysis using magnesium sulfate. Semin Perinatol 1981;5:266–73.
[27] Peaceman AM, Meyer BA, Thorp JA, et al. The effect of magnesium sulfate tocolysis on the fetal biophysical profile. Am J Obstet Gynecol 1989;161:771–4.
[28] Wright JW, Ridgway LE, Wright BD, et al. Effect of MgSO4 on heart rate monitoring in the preterm fetus. J Reprod Med 1996;41:605–8.
[29] Gray SE, Rodis JF, Lettieri L, et al. Effect of intravenous magnesium sulfate on the biophysical profile of the healthy preterm fetus. Am J Obstet Gynecol 1994;170:1131–5.

[30] Holcomb Jr WL, Shackelford GD, Petrie RH. Magnesium tocolysis and neonatal bone abnormalities: a controlled study. Obstet Gynecol 1991;78:611–4.

[31] Santi MD, Henry GW, Douglas GL. Magnesium sulfate treatment of preterm labor as a cause of abnormal neonatal bone mineralization. J Pediatr Orthop 1994;14:249–53.

[32] Lamm CI, Norton KI, Murphy RJC, et al. Congenital rickets associated with magnesium sulfate infusion for tocolysis. J Pediatr 1988;113:1078–82.

[33] Nelson KB, Grether JK. Can magnesium sulfate reduce the risk of cerebral palsy in very low birthweight infants? Pediatrics 1995;95:263–9.

[34] Hauth JC, Goldenberg RL, Nelson KG, et al. Reduction of cerebral palsy with maternal MgSO4 treatment in newborns weighing 500–1000g [abstract]. Am J Obstet Gynecol 1995; 172(1 pt 2):419.

[35] Schendel DE, Berg CJ, Yeargin-Allsopp M, et al. Prenatal magnesium sulfate exposure and the risk for cerebral palsy or mental retardation among very low-birth-weight children aged 3 to 5 years. JAMA 1996;276:1805–10.

[36] Kuban KC, Leviton A, Pagano M, et al. Maternal toxemia is associated with reduced incidence of germinal matrix hemorrhage in premature babies. J Child Neurol 1992;7:70–6.

[37] FineSmith RB, Rocke K, Yellin PB, et al. Effect of magnesium sulfate on the development of cystic periventricular leukomalacia in preterm infants. Am J Perinatol 1997;14:303–7.

[38] Grether JK, Hoogstrate J, Selvin S, et al. Magnesium sulfate tocolysis and risk of neonatal death. Am J Obstet Gynecol 1998;178:1–6.

[39] Crowther CA, Hiller JE, Doyle LW, et al. Effect of magnesium sulfate given for neuroprotection before preterm birth: a randomized controlled trial. JAMA 2003;290:2669–76.

[40] Mittendorf R, Pryde P, Khoshnood B, et al. If tocolytic magnesium sulfate is associated with excess total pediatric mortality, what is its impact? Obstet Gynecol 1998;92:308–11.

[41] Scudiero R, Khoshnood B, Pryde PG, et al. Perinatal death and tocolytic magnesium sulfate. Obstet Gynecol 2000;96:178–82.

[42] Kimberlin DF, Hauth JC, Goldenberg RL, et al. The effect of maternal magnesium sulfate treatment on neonatal morbidity in ≤1000-gram infants. Am J Perinatol 1998;15:635–41.

[43] Spisso KR, Harbert GM, Thiagarajah S. The use of magnesium sulfate as the primary tocolytic agent to prevent premature delivery. Am J Obstet Gynecol 1982;142:840–5.

[44] Taslimi MM, Sibai BM, Amon E, et al. A national survey on preterm labor. Am J Obstet Gynecol 1989;160:1352–60.

[45] Cotton DB, Strassner HT, Hill LM, et al. Comparison of magnesium sulfate, terbutaline and a placebo for inhibition of preterm labor: a randomized study. J Reprod Med 1984;29:92–7.

[46] Cox SM, Sherman ML, Leveno KJ. Randomized investigation of magnesium sulfate for prevention of preterm birth. Am J Obstet Gynecol 1990;163:767–72.

[47] Crowther CA, Hiller JE, Doyle LW. Magnesium sulphate for preventing preterm birth in threatened preterm labour. The Cochrane Database of Systematic Reviews 2002 [Issue 4. Art. No.: CD001060. DOI:10.1002/14651858.CD001060].

[48] Zuckerman H, Reiss U, Ruberstein I. The inhibition of human premature labor by indomethacin. Obstet Gynecol 1974;44:787–92.

[49] Morales WJ, Madhav H. Efficacy and safety of indomethacin compared with magnesium sulfate in the management of preterm labor: a randomized study. Am J Obstet Gynecol 1993;169: 97–102.

[50] Schorr SJ, Ascarelli MH, Rust OA, et al. A comparative study of ketorolac (Toradol) and magnesium sulfate for arrest of preterm labor. South Med J 1998;91:1028–32.

[51] McWhorter J, Carlan SJ, O'Leary TD, et al. Rofecoxib versus magnesium sulfate to arrest preterm labor: a randomized trial. Obstet Gynecol 2004;103:923–30.

[52] Glock JL, Morales WJ. Efficacy and safety of nifedipine versus magnesium sulfate in the management of preterm labor: a randomized study. Am J Obstet Gynecol 1993;169:960–4.

[53] Larmon JE, Ross BS, May WL, et al. Oral nicardipine versus intravenous magnesium sulfate for the treatment of preterm labor. Am J Obstet Gynecol 1999;181:1432–7.

[54] El-Sayed YY, Riley ET, Holbrook Jr RH, et al. Randomized comparison of intravenous

nitroglycerin and magnesium sulfate for treatment of preterm labor. Obstet Gynecol 1999; 93:79–83.

[55] Miller Jr JM, Keane MWD, Horger III EO. A comparison of magnesium sulfate and terbutaline for the arrest of premature labor: a preliminary report. J Reprod Med 1982;27:348–51.

[56] Chau AC, Gabert HA, Miller Jr JM. A prospective comparison of terbutaline and magnesium for tocolysis. Obstet Gynecol 1992;80:847–51.

[57] Wilkins IA, Lynch L, Mehalek KE, et al. Efficacy and side effects of magnesium sulfate and ritodrine as tocolytic agents. Am J Obstet Gynecol 1988;159:685–9.

[58] Beall MH, Edgar BW, Paul RH, et al. A comparison of ritodrine, terbutaline, and magnesium for the suppression of preterm labor. Am J Obstet Gynecol 1985;153:854–9.

[59] Hatjis CG. Ritodrine/magnesium for the treatment of premature labor. Am J Obstet Gynecol 1984;150:108.

[60] Hatjis CG, Swain M, Nelson LH, et al. Efficacy of combined administration of magnesium sulfate and ritodrine in the treatment of premature labor. Obstet Gynecol 1987;69:317–22.

[61] Ogburn Jr PL, Hansen CA, Williams PP, et al. Magnesium sulfate and β-mimetic dual-agent tocolysis in preterm labor after single-agent failure. J Reprod Med 1985;30:583–7.

[62] Coleman FH. Safety and efficacy of combined ritodrine and magnesium sulfate for preterm labor: a method for reduction of complications. Am J Perinatol 1990;7:366–9.

[63] Kosasa TS, Busse R, Wahl N, et al. Long-term tocolysis with combined intravenous terbutaline and magnesium sulfate: a 10-year study of 1000 patients. Obstet Gynecol 1994;84:369–73.

[64] Lewis DF, Grimshaw A, Brooks GG, et al. A comparison of magnesium sulfate and indomethacin to magnesium sulfate only for tocolysis in preterm labor with advanced cervical dilation. South Med J 1995;88:737–40.

[65] Terrone DA, Rinehart BK, Kimmel ES, et al. A prospective, randomized, controlled trial of high and low maintenance doses of magnesium sulfate for acute tocolysis. Am J Obstet Gynecol 2000;182(6):1477–82.

[66] Lewis DF, Gallaspy JW, Fontenot MT, et al. Successful tocolysis: does cervical change affect time to delivery? Am J Perinatol 1997;14:593–6.

[67] Martin RW, Gaddy DK, Martin JN, et al. Tocolysis with oral magnesium. Am J Obstet Gynecol 1987;156:433–4.

[68] Martin RW, Perry Jr KG, Hess LW, et al. Oral magnesium and the prevention of preterm labor in a high-risk group of patients. Am J Obstet Gynecol 1992;166:144–7.

[69] Garite TJ, Keegan KA, Freeman RK, et al. A randomized trial of ritodrine tocolysis versus expectant management in patients with premature rupture of membranes at 25 to 30 weeks of gestation. Am J Obstet Gynecol 1987;157:388.

[70] Fontenot T, Lewis DF. Tocolytic therapy with preterm premature rupture of membranes. Clin Perinatol 2001;28:787–96.

[71] Fortunato SJ, Welt SI, Eggleston M, et al. Prolongation of the latency period in preterm premature rupture of the membranes using prophylactic antibiotics and tocolysis. J Perinatol 1990;10:252.

[72] Matsuda Y, Ikenoue T, Hokanishi H. Premature rupture of the membranes-aggressive versus conservative approach: effect of tocolytic and antibiotic therapy. Gynecol Obstet Invest 1993; 36:102.

[73] Dudley D, Gagnon D, Varner M. Long-term tocolysis with intravenous magnesium sulfate. Obstet Gynecol 1989;73:373–8.

[74] Wilkins IA, Goldberg JD, Phillips RN, et al. Long-term use of magnesium sulfate as a tocolytic agent. Obstet Gynecol 1986;67:38S–40S.

[75] Pryde PG, Besinger RE, Gianopoulos JG, et al. Adverse and beneficial effects of tocolytic therapy. Semin Perinatol 2001;25:316–40.

[76] Lewis DF, Bergstedt S, Edwards MS, et al. Successful magnesium sulfate tocolysis: is "weaning" the drug necessary? Am J Obstet Gynecol 1997;177:742–5.

ELSEVIER
SAUNDERS

Obstet Gynecol Clin N Am
32 (2005) 501–517

OBSTETRICS AND
GYNECOLOGY
CLINICS
OF NORTH AMERICA

Antiprostaglandin Drugs

Stephen T. Vermillion, MD*, Christopher J. Robinson, MD

*Division of Maternal Fetal Medicine, Department of Obstetrics and Gynecology,
Medical University of South Carolina, 96 Jonathan Lucas Street, Suite 634, PO Box 250619,
Charleston, SC 29425, USA*

Despite continued efforts aimed at preterm birth prevention, as many as 12% of all deliveries in the United States are preterm. Even more staggering is the fact that prematurity in and of itself accounts for more than 85% of all the perinatal morbidity and mortality [1,2]. Unfortunately, additional evidence indicates that the incidence of preterm birth is on a steady upward trend as demonstrated by the fact that from 1992 to 2002 the rate increased from 10.2% to 12.1% [3]. Stated in economic terms, the direct and indirect costs for the sequelae of preterm birth have been estimated between $6 to $10 billon dollars annually.

Preterm birth should more appropriately be classified as a syndrome because of the complex, multifactorial nature of this disorder [4]. The primary intervention for preterm labor remains tocolytic therapy aimed at prolongation of gestation with the primary focus of allowing sufficient time for administration of antenatal corticosteroids. In arresting preterm labor, many tocolytics with varying mechanisms of action have been used. One of the most efficacious tocolytic therapies used to date is indomethacin, an antiprostaglandin drug. This article reviews the evidence for antiprostaglandin agents as tocolytic therapy, providing practitioners with guidelines for clinical use.

Antiprostaglandin drugs: mechanism of action

Antiprostaglandin agents arrest labor through the inhibition of the enzyme prostaglandin synthetase or cyclooxygenase (COX). This enzyme is responsible for the conversion of arachidonic acid to an intermediate endoperoxide and

---

* Corresponding author.
E-mail address: vermills@musc.edu (S.T. Vermillion).

finally resulting in the formation of a prostaglandin. Prostaglandins are 20-carbon fatty acid chains that function as hormones and are produced constitutively in most cells of the body. The biologically active forms are derived from arachidonic acid, which is a common component of most cellular membranes. The initial step in the formation of prostaglandins involves the liberation of arachidonic acid by phospholipases from the phospholipid bi-layer of the cell membrane. Next, arachidonic acid is reduced by COX to form an unstable intermediate endoperoxide (prostaglandin G_2). This unstable intermediate is then converted to prostacyclin, thromboxane, or prostaglandins E_2 or $F_{2\alpha}$. Given that prostaglandins E_2 or $F_{2\alpha}$ are involved in preterm labor and parturition (preterm or term), the inhibition of their synthesis is an appropriate pharmacologic target in the reduction of preterm deliveries [5]. Antiprostaglandin drugs act by inhibiting COX activity and thereby blocking the conversion of arachidonic acid to prostaglandin precursors (Fig. 1).

Normal parturition has been described to occur in four distinct, hormonally modulated phases: (1) functional quiescence, (2) activation, (3) stimulation, and (4) involution [6]. Quiescence represents the baseline resting uterine tone found in a normal pregnancy before onset of labor. Less is understood about the mechanisms that transform this quiescent tone into the activation phase of parturition. Activation represents the priming of the uterus to enter the stimulation phase of labor where coordinated myometrial activity occurs and leads to phasic uterine contractions and delivery. Involution follows the delivery of the fetus and returns the uterus to its prepregnancy state. Mechanisms behind parturition have been studied and explained in animal models but none of these have been extrapolated to fully understand human parturition. Prostaglandins have been identified as key components in the process of both normal and preterm labor. First, prostaglandins are facilitators of myometrial contractions by increases in calcium within myometrial cells leading to increased activity of myosin light chain kinase, a protein directly tied to myometrial contraction. This initial activity of prostaglandins leads to increased myometrial activity in the form of isolated cellular contractions that ultimately must become coordinated such that a sufficient combined force is developed effectively to initiate cervical change. Prostaglandins also play an important role in the coordination of contraction

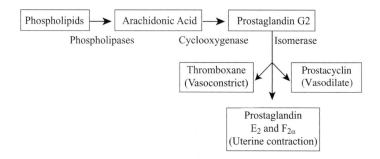

Fig. 1. Prostaglandin production.

efforts by increasing the number of gap junctions between individual myometrial cells leading to organized synchronous activity with a propulsive force [7]. Finally, prostaglandins are vital in the production of collagenases and proteases that promote ripening of the cervix [8].

Given the many roles of prostaglandins in creating conditions favorable for activation and stimulation of labor, it is readily apparent that an effective target for the prevention of preterm labor should include a focus of the inhibition of prostaglandin production. An ideal tocolytic therapy would target the prostaglandin-mediated mechanism of labor activation while not interfering with fetal development or causing undue maternal symptomatology. Additionally, it has been well studied that there are many factors that influence the endogenous formation of prostaglandins in the human body. Maternal or fetal stress, through activation of the maternal-fetal adrenal axis, is recognized to increase prostaglandin production through both corticotrophin-releasing hormone and placentally produced estrogens [5,9]. Further, investigators have demonstrated that myometrial stretching also augments prostaglandin formation through increased COX activity [10]. Finally, a hereditary deficiency of prostaglandin dehydrogenase, an enzyme involved in the metabolism of prostaglandins, may result in a basal elevation of prostaglandins in certain individuals and lead to idiopathic premature labor [6].

As this evidence suggests, prostaglandins may be the single most significant factor in the promotion of preterm labor. This realization led to interest in the use of such nonsteroidal anti-inflammatory drugs (NSAIDs) in blocking the production of prostaglandins. In 1971, Vane [11] first reported that aspirin and indomethacin block the production of prostaglandins E_2 and $F_{2\alpha}$. Given this novel pharmacologic therapy and the recognition of prostaglandin influence over labor, an immediate interest was spawned investigating indomethacin and its use in inhibiting COX to arrest preterm labor.

Cyclooxygenase specificity

There are two recognized COX enzymes, simply identified as COX-1 and COX-2 enzymes. Both of these enzymes are directly responsible for the formation of the intermediate prostaglandin G_2. These enzymes are very similar in their primary amino acid sequence, sharing approximately 65% identity [12]. COX-2 differs by the addition of 18 amino acids on the C-terminal end, however, which is thought to mediate the binding of the enzyme to the endoplasmic reticulum and may predispose the enzyme to rapid degradation [13,14]. The x-ray crystallography structures of the two COX enzyme isoforms are nearly identical except for a critical amino acid exchange in a side binding pocket. Using this alteration between the COX enzymes, pharmacologists have exploited the single exchange to guide development of COX-2–specific NSAIDS. A number of pharmacologic agents have been developed to access selectively the binding site on COX-2 and inhibit its action. As expected, however, these agents do exhibit cross-reactivity between the COX isotypes and may differ in their relative potential selectively to target the inhibition of COX-2.

Selective expression of cyclooxygenase isotypes

The best known difference in the COX isotypes lies in their differential expression in different cell types. COX-1 is known to be expressed in most if not all cell types. COX-2 is found in varying levels among different tissues, however, and is usually expressed in response to the production and release of cytokines, growth factors, or various promoters. It has been well described that the expression of COX-1 is constant throughout gestation, whereas COX-2 expression increases significantly as the pregnancy progresses. Specifically, COX-2 mRNA is 100-fold higher than COX-1 mRNA at term and further doubles with onset of labor suggesting a potential role on COX-2 in normal parturition.

Numerous NSAIDS have entered the market in the past four decades including aspirin, ibuprofen, indomethacin, celecoxib, and rofecoxib. The latter two of these drugs are recognized as COX-2 selective. Given the widespread use of these medications, a host of data is available on the safety and efficacy of these drugs in treating pain and many disease processes. The selection of certain drugs may prove beneficial because of the differing pharmacologic properties of each of these drugs. The most investigated of these in preterm labor is indomethacin, where a host of data on safety and efficacy for tocolysis exists.

Pharmacokinetics of indomethacin

Indomethacin, probably the most commonly used tocolytic in this class, has been evaluated extensively to determine the pharmacology and pharmacokinetics in both the mother and fetus. Indomethacin acts by nonspecific inhibition of both of the COX-1 and COX-2 enzymes, which are essential for the conversion of arachidonic acid and fatty acids into prostaglandin endoperoxides. This inhibition is readily reversible once serum drug levels decline after discontinuation of therapy. The role of prostaglandins in the initiation and maintenance of human labor has been previously presented in detail. In brief, prostaglandins stimulate the influx of calcium ions into the uterine smooth muscle cell. Calcium then facilitates the interaction of the myosin-actin complex resulting in myocyte contraction. Additionally, prostaglandins enhance the development of gap junctions within the myometrium that coordinate myometrial activity allowing synchronized contractions. The ability of indomethacin to suppress the production of prostaglandins is the basis of its ability to inhibit preterm labor. Prostaglandins, however, have many additional functions in maintaining the normal physiology of the fetus and newborn including potent vasodilatory and vasoconstrictive effects, which are particularly important for the preservation of adequate blood flow through the developing fetal circulation [15,16]. Animal studies also indicate that prostaglandins inhibit the effect of antidiuretic hormone on the collecting duct of the fetal kidney [17]. Suppression of circulating prostaglandins from tocolysis with indomethacin may lead not only to cessation of uterine activity, but also may result in vasoconstriction and reduction in the effective blood flow to various fetal organs. This vasoconstriction is reversible after cessation of short-term use of the medication, but prolonged exposure to indomethacin may result in persistent changes in the fetal ductus arteriosus and the developing fetal cerebral and mesenteric circulations. These changes may potentially place the preterm neonate at increased risk for intraventricular hemorrhage (IVH) or bowel ischemia. Furthermore, prolonged suppression of endogenous prostaglandins may cause a decrease in the production of fetal urine and ultimately lead to oligohydramnios. Short courses of indomethacin therapy defined as less than 72 hours do not seem to promote such clinical risks [18,19].

Indomethacin can be administered by oral, rectal, or vaginal routes. Depending on the route of administration, peak maternal plasma concentrations are achieved within 2 hours after dosing with a mean half-life in the maternal serum of approximately 4.5 hours [20]. Most of the drug is metabolized by the liver but 20% to 30% is excreted in the urine unchanged. Indomethacin readily crosses the placenta with fetal umbilical artery serum concentrations equilibrating with the maternal serum levels within 5 hours of dosing [21]. The half-life in preterm neonates is approximately five times longer than that seen in the adult. The persistence of indomethacin in the serum of the fetus for a prolonged period following cessation of therapy is likely caused by the immature fetal livers ability to conjugate the active drug. Given this rapid diffusion to the fetus in concentrations equal to that in maternal serum, one must consider the drugs effect on fetal development and consequences from drug exposure. Most reports have used a 50- to 100-mg loading dose usually by rectal suppository, followed by 25 mg orally every 6 to 8 hours. Identifying the lowest effective dose is important to decrease the risk of associated side effects. The drug is contraindicated in those patients with a history of peptic ulcer disease, kidney or liver disease, hematologic abnormalities, or those with a hypersensitivity to NSAIDs. Indomethacin also has antipyretic properties; use in the setting of suspected chorioamnionitis should be cautioned because of the potential for masking a rise in maternal temperature from subclinical infection.

Indomethacin efficacy as a tocolytic

The tocolytic efficacy of indomethacin has generally been acknowledged despite the lack of large randomized trials. Several studies have compared indomethacin with placebo for the treatment of preterm labor. All the trials were limited by small sample sizes, and by the use of rescue tocolysis in those patients considered to be tocolytic failures [22,23]. Niebyl and colleagues [22] designed the first prospective randomized, double blind, placebo-controlled trial of indomethacin for preterm labor tocolysis. Thirty patients were enrolled and equally randomized based on entry criteria that required cervical change during observation or a cervix at least 2 cm dilated with contractions measured by external tocodynamometry less than 5 minutes apart. Patients were excluded if their cervix was 4 cm or more at enrollment. These investigators demonstrated that patients treated for 24 hours with indomethacin had significantly fewer deliveries within 48 hours of treatment compared with the placebo group. Success was short-lived, however, because no difference in the overall delivery rate was detected after 48 hours. Zuckerman and colleagues [23] reported slightly better success in delaying preterm delivery in a group of patients treated for 24 hours with indomethacin. Patients in the treatment group had fewer deliveries within 1 week of treatment compared with placebo controls.

Panter and colleagues [24] performed a randomized controlled trial of indomethacin versus placebo that enrolled 34 patients for the cessation of preterm labor. Despite the fact that only 3 of 16 patients in the indomethacin arm delivered within 48 hours compared with 8 of 18 patients in the placebo arm, this difference because of the limited sample size was not considered to be statistically significant. Finally, a systematic review combining these three trials for improved statistical power was performed [25]. In this analysis the investigators successfully were able to demonstrate a significant reduction in the number of patients delivering within 48 hours in the group treated with indomethacin. Ultimately, however, investigators were unable to demonstrate a difference in neonatal outcomes between the treatment and control groups. Interpreting the efficacy of tocolytic agents in preterm labor trials is difficult because of the heterogenous definitions used to describe success. Prolonging pregnancy for at least 48 hours may allow for the benefit of corticosteroid administration; however, if neonatal outcomes are unchanged then success is difficult to claim.

Other trials have reported similar efficacy and fewer maternal side effects when comparing indomethacin with betamimetics [26,27]. Ultimately, despite the prolongation of gestation and cessation of preterm labor, these investigations too were unable to demonstrate a neonatal benefit following tocolysis. These trials were also limited by small sample sizes that were inadequate to assess neonatal outcomes. Recognizing these limitations, several investigators have evaluated the efficacy of indomethacin compared with other tocolytic agents by performing two separate systematic reviews of available randomized controlled trials. Keirse [28] established that indomethacin was successful at reducing delivery within 48 hours and before 37 weeks, and decreasing the frequency of low–birth weight births. These authors were unable to demonstrate a significant reduction in the frequencies of respiratory distress syndrome and fetal or neonatal death. Similarly, Gyetvai and colleagues [29] reported that indomethacin reduced delivery within 48 hours, reduced delivery within 7 days, and reduced deliveries before 37 weeks' gestation. Compared with betamimetics, magnesium sulfate, atosiban, and ethanol, indomethacin proved superior in tocolytic efficacy without an increase in neonatal or maternal morbidity or mortality.

Fetal and neonatal complications associated with indomethacin

Tocolytic therapy with indomethacin has been associated with several potentially significant fetal and neonatal complications in a number of reports (Box 1). Most of these cited complications were associated with prolonged administration with little or no fetal surveillance. The most widely reported complication associated with antenatal exposure to indomethacin is constriction of fetal ductus arteriosus. This association was suspected because of the ability of indomethacin to close the persistently patent ductus arteriosus in the newborn period. Animal studies have specifically identified COX-1–dependent prostaglandins as the predominant mediators of ductal patency in utero [30]. Because of its nonselective nature, indomethacin inhibits both COX-1 and COX-2 enzymes. A few early investigations reported isolated cases of primary pulmonary hypertension in the newborn after prolonged in utero exposure to indomethacin presumably caused by prolonged constriction of fetal ductus arteriosus [27,31,32]. Prolonged shunting of blood away from the constricted ductus arteriosus and through the pulmonary vasculature is believed to lead to hypertrophy of the muscular walls of the pulmonary vessels.

Closer evaluation of the effect of extended tocolysis with indomethacin on the developing fetal ductus arteriosus has demonstrated increased sensitivity of the ductus to indomethacin with advancing gestation. Moise [33] was the first to evaluate the developing fetal ductus arteriosus with serial fetal echocardiography. Moise demonstrated that fetuses exposed to indomethacin had a significant increase in the frequency of ductal constriction around 32 weeks' gestation. Using a similar study protocol at their institution, the authors followed 72 fetuses exposed in utero to prolonged courses (> 48–72 hours) of indomethacin [34]. Although 70% of the fetuses that developed ductal constriction in that study did so around 32 weeks, there were several cases of ductal constriction that occurred at earlier gestational ages, even as early as 25 weeks.

The study protocols used in the two studies described previously have served as the basis for the current recommendations for monitoring patients receiving antenatal indomethacin (Boxes 2 and 3). Initially, indomethacin therapy should be limited to gestations less than 32 weeks because of the increasing likelihood of

---

Box 1. Potential indomethacin-associated fetal and neonatal complications

Fetal ductus arteriosus constriction
Intraventricular hemorrhage
Necrotizing enterocolitis
Oliguria
Oligohydramnios
Persistent neonatal patent ductus arteriosus

Box 2. Prevention of complications from indomethacin tocolysis

Restrict usage to <32 weeks' gestation
Limit duration of therapy to less than 72 hours if possible
Avoid treatment with growth-restricted fetuses
Avoid therapy in the setting of oligohydramnios

---

ductal constriction to develop after this gestational age. After 48 to 72 hours of therapy, if the decision is made to continue treatment with indomethacin, then fetal echocardiography should be performed to detect any evidence of ductal constriction. Ductal constriction is evidenced by increasing ductal blood flow velocities (systolic >1.4 m/s, diastolic >0.35 m/s) and in some cases by the appearance of tricuspid valve regurgitation [33,34]. All fetuses should be individually evaluated in the case of multiple gestations because variations in ductal flow velocities can exist between fetuses of the same pregnancy. If normal ductal flow velocities are identified, then echocardiographic evaluations should be repeated weekly for the duration of the therapy. Fetal echocardiography is not necessary if the decision has been made to discontinue therapy. Approximately 50% of the fetuses in the authors' study using maintenance indomethacin tocolysis developed mild ductal constriction at some point; however, all of these cases demonstrated complete resolution of the constriction with prompt discontinuation of the therapy [34]. Therapy should be discontinued in all cases of constriction. If increasing but not abnormal ductal flow velocities are identified, dosing may be tapered from every 6 hours to 8- or 12-hour dosing intervals with repeat echocardiography performed within 24 to 48 hours. Patients receiving only

---

Box 3. Fetal surveillance with maintenance tocolysis using indomethacin

Fetal echocardiography for the detection of ductal constriction

Initially after 48–72 hours of therapy
Weekly for the duration of tocolysis
Discontinue therapy if constriction detected

Amniotic fluid evaluation for the detection of oligohydramnios

Before initiating therapy
After 48–72 hours of therapy
Twice weekly for the duration of tocolysis
Discontinue therapy if oligohydramnios detected

---

a short course (<72 hours) of indomethacin do not need echocardiographic evaluation because of the inherent reversibility of fetal ductal constriction.

Less clear is the surveillance needed for intermittent short courses of indomethacin. Based on pharmacologic data it seems reasonable to defer ductal evaluation if the interval between treatment courses is greater than 48 hours. Indomethacin should be avoided in pregnancies complicated by intrauterine growth restriction because of the potential for ductal constriction and possible perfusion abnormalities.

Indomethacin has also been used for the treatment of symptomatic poly-hydramnios because of its ability to cause a diminution of the amniotic fluid volume within a few days [35]. Recognizing this effect, amniotic fluid volume measurements should be evaluated twice weekly for evidence of developing oligohydramnios. Indomethacin should be discontinued or tapered with any trend toward oligohydramnios. Oligohydramnios developed in about 10% of pregnancies in the authors' study of maintenance tocolysis with indomethacin [34]. All of these cases had complete normalization of the amniotic fluid volume after prompt discontinuation of treatment.

In a retrospective review, Norton and colleagues [36] reported an increase in the frequency of advanced-grade IVH in preterm infants after indomethacin tocolysis. Limitations of that study included marked variation in the medication dosing and surveillance regimens. Additionally, the increased risk of advanced-grade IVH reported in that study was the result of the inclusion of grade II IVH along with the more clinically significant grades III to IV. Only grade II IVH was significantly associated with indomethacin exposure, whereas grades III to IV were similar between the treatment and control groups. Some have hypothesized that the development of IVH after indomethacin tocolysis may actually be associated with prolonged constriction of the ductus. Ductal constriction increases the shunting of blood through the fetal carotids resulting in alterations in cerebral perfusion, which may predispose the premature infant to IVH. Echocardiographic evaluation of the fetal ductus arteriosus was not routinely incorporated into the Norton study so it is not possible to comment specifically on the potential association of IVH with ductal constriction.

To evaluate the potential risks associated with antenatal exposure to indomethacin further, the authors performed a case control study of 75 infants exposed to at least 24 hours of indomethacin within 72 hours of delivery occurring before 32 weeks' gestation [37]. The neonatal outcomes of these infants were compared with 150 infants matched for gestational age, mode of delivery, fetal sex, and race. Overall, the indomethacin-exposed neonates experienced no increase on any measure of neonatal morbidity. Interestingly, a trend toward a reduction in advanced-grade IVH was found in those neonates recently exposed to a short course of antenatal indomethacin. A protective effect of low-dose indomethacin administered during the first 72 hours of life to very low–birth weight infants against IVH has been reported [38]. Perhaps limited doses of indomethacin administered shortly before delivery may provide similar prophylactic effects, although further studies are needed to explore this possibility.

Several studies have demonstrated that premature newborns have an increased frequency of persistent patent ductus arteriosus unresponsive to medical management after antenatal indomethacin tocolysis [36,39]. It is logical that suppression of vasodilatory prostaglandins with indomethacin could cause constriction of the fetal ductus arteriosus. Less convincing, however, is the association of persistent patent ductus in the newborn with antenatal indomethacin exposure. The theory is that a secondary compensatory surge in prostaglandin production occurs after discontinuation of indomethacin therapy. This surge results in supranormal prostaglandin concentrations after delivery causing protracted vasodilatation of the ductus. Recent antenatal exposure seems to be the most significant risk factor in these studies, although the authors' recent study has not shown this association [37].

Constriction or closure of the fetal ductus following indomethacin tocolysis led to concerns over how the resultant altered fetal cardiovascular physiology might also alter central nervous system or renal perfusion. Isolated case reports of fetal renal failure and IVH had been reported in neonates born following indomethacin tocolysis [40,41]. Mari and colleagues [42] investigated the pulsatility index of the middle cerebral artery in fetuses both before and during indomethacin tocolysis to determine whether ductal constriction alters cerebral circulation. In this study, 11 fetuses developed ductal constriction within 48 hours of onset of indomethacin tocolysis and rapidly reversed within 48 hours following cessation of therapy. Of the fetuses with ductal constriction, those without tricuspid regurgitation had no change in middle cerebral artery pulsatility index. In four fetuses with both ductal constriction and tricuspid regurgitation, however, a significant difference was observed in middle cerebral artery pulsatility indexes (2.22 versus 1.57, $P < .05$). No adverse neonatal outcomes were reported in either group. This investigation was followed by a randomized comparison of middle cerebral artery resistance index both before and during either magnesium or indomethacin tocolysis [43]. In this trial, 12 patients were randomized to each group and no significant differences were seen in middle cerebral artery flow between fetuses receiving indomethacin or magnesium tocolysis. Again, this study also demonstrated no change in the resistive index while on therapy as compared with baseline measurements. These investigators also noted no significant difference in the rate of IVH between magnesium- or indomethacin-exposed fetuses.

Two studies have focused on the possibility of an increased risk for neonatal complications if delivery occurs within 48 hours of indomethacin exposure. Souter and coworkers [39] reported that neonates delivered after recent tocolysis with indomethacin were at an increased risk for developing IVH [39]. Many patients in this study, however, received prolonged indomethacin therapy with limited fetal surveillance. Also, patients with premature rupture of the membranes were included in the cohort, which may have increased the overall frequency of IVH caused by infectious causes. No increased neonatal risks were identified in those infants delivered more than 48 hours after the last dose of indomethacin. Major and colleagues [44] demonstrated that neonates delivered within 24 to

48 hours of antenatal indomethacin exposure were more likely to be diagnosed with necrotizing enterocolitis. Similar to the study by Souter and coworkers [39], patients who received prolonged treatment with indomethacin were included. Recognizing the concern for recent indomethacin exposure and subsequent neonatal complications, the authors evaluated the effect of short-term indomethacin tocolysis in those neonates that ultimately failed tocolysis and delivered within 72 hours of exposure [37]. They were unable to demonstrate a significant difference in the frequency of necrotizing enterocolitis, persistent patent ductus arteriosus, or IVH after recent indomethacin exposure compared with matched controls. The duration of therapy with indomethacin is a more significant risk factor than is the timing of exposure.

Cyxlooxygenase-2 inhibitors: rationale and use in preterm labor

The development of COX-2–specific inhibitors has provided a safer alternative to traditional NSAIDs. They are effective as analgesics with decreased incidence of gastrointestinal ulcerative complications, and there is an increasing body of evidence that they may be effective in reducing the incidence of colorectal carcinomas [45]. Recently, the potential for use as a tocolytic has been examined.

As indomethacin, a nonselective COX-1–COX-2 inhibitor, became recognized as a potent inhibitor of preterm labor, it remained mostly a second-line tocolytic therapy because of the potential fetal and neonatal complications that had been described with its use. Understanding that COX-1 is an enzyme expressed in most fetal tissues, the blockade of this enzyme could easily affect many fetal organ systems while exerting tocolytic effect. COX-1 enzyme expression had been previously described in the ductus arteriosus, fetal kidneys, and fetal gastrointestinal tract. Notably, each of these organ systems had been reported to be involved in complications following indomethacin tocolysis. Given a basic desire of therapy to ameliorate preterm labor without undue fetal complication, COX-2–selective inhibitors have been investigated in animal and human preterm labor in hopes of ascertaining an understanding of their efficacy and monitoring for potential complications.

The interest in COX-2–selective inhibition of preterm labor was prefaced by both bench research and animal studies conducted to exhibit biologic plausibility and safety. First, both COX-1 and COX-2 expression were verified in the chorion, amnion, placenta, and fetal tissues. It was noted that up-regulation of COX-2 was responsible for the increased prostaglandin synthesis at term. Furthermore, the expression of COX-1 in these tissues remained stable throughout pregnancy, whereas COX-2 was increasingly expressed as gestation progressed. The most notable increase in COX-2 was identified in the second trimester with an exponential increase throughout the third trimester peaking at delivery. Following delivery, the expression of COX-2 in the decidua was found to regress to similar expression levels of COX-1. Considering these data, COX-2 seemed to play an integral role in the fetomaternal structures, whereas COX-1 seemed to be unaffected by pregnancy [46].

Cyxlooxygenase-2 inhibitors: safety

Further excitement was generated for COX-2 inhibitors as tocolytics following the description of differential expression in human fetal models. Again, these models demonstrated a constitutive expression of COX-1 in fetal lung, kidney, and intestine. Also, the fetal ductus arteriosus closure was described as being greatly mediated by COX-1–induced prostaglandin synthesis. These findings suggested that COX-2–selective agents may be effective tocolytics while avoiding the adverse fetal effect of ductal constriction. This initial excitement was tempered, however, when COX-2 was subsequently demonstrated to be up-regulated with advancing gestational age in each of these tissues [47]. This presented a potential difficulty, because it is uncertain as to whether the selective inhibition of COX-2 affects the development of these fetal organs.

The COX-2 inhibitors nimesulide, celecoxib, and rofecoxib have about 15, 375, and 800 times greater affinity for the COX-2 subtype, respectively [48]. When given to pregnant lambs, celecoxib caused constriction of the ductus arteriosus, but to a significantly less degree than indomethacin [49]. When administered to newborn pigs, a COX-2 inhibitor did not affect the ductus, whereas a COX-1 inhibitor caused as much constriction as indomethacin [30].

Complications of prematurity, such as necrotizing enterocolitis and IVH, may be increased with concurrent indomethacin [36]. It has been suggested that this finding is the result of a concurrent risk factor [50]. Cases of preterm labor recalcitrant to first-line tocolysis, most often magnesium sulfate, are more likely to have an intra-amniotic infection [51]. Unfortunately, these are the cases requiring indomethacin use. Intra-amniotic infection alone increases necrotizing enterocolitis and IVH, possibly laying undue blame on indomethacin. It has been proposed that if indomethacin increases the risk of IVH, it is because of inhibition of platelet aggregation. COX-2 inhibitors do not have antiplatelet activity, and should not increase this risk unless an additional mechanism is at play [48]. The mechanism of necrotizing enterocolitis is under investigation. If phospholipids, arachidonic acid, or its metabolites play a role, as has been suggested [52], NSAIDs would certainly be involved. Whether COX-2 inhibitors would be protective, have no effect, or be detrimental remains to be seen.

COX-2 inhibitors impair development of the renal cortex, decreasing the diameter of the glomerulus in mice and rats when given throughout gestation [53]. In selected case reports, infants of women taking COX-2 inhibitors have been born with renal damage, both end-stage and transient type [54,55]. These clinical outcomes were primarily seen outside the United States with the use of nimesulide, however, which has much less specificity for COX-2 than celecoxib and rofecoxib and is often referred to as a "COX-2–selective inhibitor," rather than a "COX-2–specific inhibitor." Furthermore, its use was often continued beyond the preterm period. If inhibition of COX-2 has significant in utero renal effects, it may be responsible for the decrease in amniotic fluid volume associated with indomethacin use, both as a side effect and as a primary treatment outcome [56]. The renal effects when exposed to COX-2 inhibitors during the short window from viability to near term need to be examined.

More recently and more promising, the COX-2 inhibitor meloxicam has been studied to assess whether administration of the medication in sheep models induced any changes in COX protein expression in different fetal tissues [57]. These authors reported no significant change in COX-1 or COX-2 protein expression in fetal kidney, lung, small intestine, adrenal gland, heart, liver, or brain tissues when compared with saline controls. The authors speculated that meloxicam, when used at the studied doses, may be a promising tocolytic agent in this class because of the potential to avoid fetal complications with its use.

The safety of celecoxib has been compared with indomethacin in one small but very compelling randomized control trial that evaluated the short-term use (48 hours) of each agent in 24 pregnant women presenting with preterm labor between 24 and 34 weeks gestation [58]. Women were randomized to receive either 100 mg of celecoxib orally every 12 hours or 100-mg indomethacin suppository followed by 50 mg orally every 6 hours, both for a total of 48 hours. Fetal surveillance included a baseline ultrasound assessment of amniotic fluid index, deepest vertical amniotic fluid pocket, fetal ductus arteriosus velocity measurements by Doppler to assess the patency and constriction of the vessel, and subjective evaluation of the fetal tricuspid valve for regurgitant flow consistent with ductal constriction. This was repeated at 24-hour intervals for 72 hours after initiation of the study drug. Interestingly, these investigators were able demonstrate a significant reduction in the amniotic fluid index in the indomethacin-treated group, which was evident within 24 hours of treatment initiation. Additionally, the mean maximum ductal velocities were significantly elevated at 24 and 72 hours in the indomethacin group when compared with the celecoxib-treated fetuses. Despite the modest increase in velocity in the indomethacin group, only one fetus exhibited measurements and findings consistent with ductal stenosis. Additionally, none of the fetuses in the celecoxib group had any significant changes in ductal velocity over the baseline measurements.

Cyxlooxygenase-2 inhibitors: efficacy as a tocolytic

In vitro studies of COX-2 inhibitors have successfully demonstrated an effective tocolytic potential. One of these evaluations used three inhibitors: (1) nimesulide, (2) meloxicam, and (3) celecoxib. Myometrial strips were derived from women during term elective or intrapartum cesarean sections. In this trial, all three inhibitors demonstrated efficacy in arresting oxytocin-induced myometrial activity [59].

Human trials have used a number of COX-2 inhibitors with differing selectivity for specific inhibition. Most of these experiments, however, were with only a few patients in pilot studies with novel, but limited results. McWhorter and colleagues [60] performed on of the largest randomized trials to date comparing oral rofecoxib with parenteral magnesium for acute tocolysis efficacy and safety. In this study, 214 patients presenting with preterm labor between 22 and 34 weeks' gestation were randomized to receive either 50 mg of rofecoxib orally or intravenous magnesium for 48 hours. The outcomes studied included delay of delivery for 48 hours and the incidence of side effects. These authors reported that delivery was delayed for 48 hours in 90% and 88% of participants in the rofecoxib and magnesium groups, respectively. The investigators did comment of the fact that there was difference between the groups in advancement of cervical dilation digitally, shortening of cervical length by transvaginal sonography, measured differences in amniotic fluid volumes, or differences in neonatal outcomes during the study period. There was greater reported incidence of maternal side effects in the magnesium group with lethargy being the most common complaint. Although the study sample size is quite large, the statistical analysis revealed a significant shortfall in power to make a decisive negative conclusion.

Cyxlooxygenase-2 inhibitors: new safety concerns

Despite the promising efforts demonstrating COX-2 safety and efficacy as tocolytic agents, the recent emergence of safety issues with COX-2 inhibitors in the nonpregnant population is an obvious concern. Several large trials have suggested an increased risk for cardiovascular complications, especially in certain populations using various COX-2 agents chronically. It is premature to assume that these medications offer no benefit in obstetrics because of these emerging data. It should be highlighted that the populations studied were older and many with underlying cardiac or other serious chronic diseases, which is significantly different than the relative health of an obstetric population in comparison. There are hopes that with further research using healthier populations that these concerns will be limited to select populations. Until then, an exercise of caution is recommended with COX-2 use in the pregnant population until further studies clarify these potential risks.

References

[1] Rush RW, Keirse MJ, Howat P, et al. Contribution of preterm birth to perinatal mortality. BMJ 1976;1976:965–8.
[2] Moutquin JM. Classification and heterogeneity of preterm birth. Br J Obstet Gynaecol 2003; 110(Suppl 20):23–30.
[3] March of Dimes. Born too soon and too small in the United States. Available at: www. marchofdimes.com. Accessed April 1, 2005.
[4] Villar J, Ezcurra EJ, de la Fuente VJ, et al. Pre-term delivery syndrome: the unmet need. Res Clin Forums 1994;16:9–33.
[5] Weiss G. Endocrinology of parturition. J Clin Endocrinol Metab 2000;85:4421–5.

[6] Challis JRG, Gibb W. Control of parturition. Prenat Neonat Med 1996;1:283–91.

[7] Garfield RE, Blennerhassett MG, Miller SM. Control of myometrial contractility: role and regulation of gap junctions. Oxf Rev Reprod Biol 1988;10:436–90.

[8] Rath W, Adelmann-Grill BC, Pieper U, et al. The role of collagenases and proteases in prostaglandin-induced cervical ripening. Prostaglandins 1987;34:119–27.

[9] Lockwood CJ. Stress-associated preterm delivery: the role of corticotropin-releasing hormone. Am J Obstet Gynecol 1999;180:S264–6.

[10] Kanayama N, Fukamizu H. Mechanical stretching increases prostaglandin E2 in cultured human amnion cells. Gynecol Obstet Invest 1989;28:123–8.

[11] Vane JR. Inhibition of prostaglandin synthesis as a mechanism of action for aspirin like drugs. Nat New Biol 1971;231:232–5.

[12] Xie WL, Chipman JG, Robertson DL, et al. Expression of a mitogen-responsive gene encoding prostaglandin synthase is regulated by mRNA splicing. Proc Natl Acad Sci U S A 1991;88: 2692–6.

[13] Spencer AG, Thuresson E, Otto JC, et al. The membrane binding domains of prostaglandin endoperoxide H synthases 1 and 2. J Biol Chem 1999;274:32936–42.

[14] Otto JC, Smith WL. Photolabeling of prostaglandin endoperoxide H synthase-1 with 3-trifluoro-3-(m-[125I]iodophenyl)diazirine as a probe of membrane association and the cyclooxygenase active site. J Biol Chem 1996;271:9906–10.

[15] Cassin S. Role of prostaglandins, thromboxanes, and leukotrienes in the control of the pulmonary circulation in the fetus and newborn. Semin Perinatol 1980;4:23–8.

[16] Clyman RI. Ontogeny of the ductus arteriosus response to prostaglandins and inhibitors of their synthesis. Semin Perinatol 1980;4:115–24.

[17] Anderson RJ, Berl T, McDonald KM, et al. Evidence for an in vivo antagonism between vasopressin and prostaglandin in the mammalian kidney. J Clin Invest 1975;56:420–6.

[18] Moise KL, Huhta JC, Sharif DS, et al. Indomethacin in the treatment of premature labor: effects on the fetal ductus arteriosis. N Engl J Med 1988;319:327–31.

[19] Vermillion ST, Scardo JA, Lashus AG, et al. The effect of indomethacin tocolysis on fetal ductus arteriosus constriction with advancing gestational age. Am J Obstet Gynecol 1997;177:256–9 [discussion: 259–61].

[20] Alvan G, Orne M, Bertilsson L, et al. Pharmacokinetics of indomethacin. Clin Pharmacol Ther 1976;18:364–73.

[21] Bhat R, Vidyasager D, Vadapalli MO, et al. Disposition of indomethacin in preterm infants. J Pediatr 1979;95:313–6.

[22] Niebyl JR, Blake DA, White RD, et al. The inhibition of premature labor with indomethacin. Am J Obstet Gynecol 1980;136:1014–9.

[23] Zuckerman H, Shalev E, Gilad G, et al. Further study of the inhibition of premature labor by indomethacin. J Perinat Med 1984;12:25–9.

[24] Panter K, Hannah M, Amankwa K, et al. The effect of indomethacin tocolysis in preterm labour on perinatal outcome: a randomized placebo-controlled trial. Br J Obstet Gynaecol 1999;106: 467–73.

[25] Mitchell BF, Olson DM. Prostaglandin endoperoxide H synthase inhibitors and other tocolytics in preterm labour. Prostaglandins Leukot Essent Fatty Acids 2004;70:167–87.

[26] Besinger R, Niebyl J, Keyes WG, et al. Randomized comparative trial of indomethacin and ritodrine for the long term treatment of preterm labor. Am J Obstet Gynecol 1991;164:981–7.

[27] Morales WJ, Smith SG, Angel JL, et al. Efficacy and safety of indomethacin versus ritodrine in the management of preterm labor: a randomized study. Obstet Gynecol 1989;74:567–72.

[28] Keirse M. Indomethacin tocolysis in preterm labour. In: Enkin M, Keirse M, Renfrew J, et al, editors. Pregnancy and childbirth module of the Cochrane Database of Systematic Reviews. London: BMJ Publishing Group; 1995.

[29] Gyetvai K, Hannah M, Hodnett E, et al. Tocolytics for preterm labor: a systematic review. Obstet Gynecol 1999;94:869–77.

[30] Guerguerian AM, Hardy P, Bhattacharya M, et al. Expression of cyclooxygenases in ductus arteriosus of fetal and newborn pigs. Am J Obstet Gynecol 1998;179:1618–26.

[31] Manchester D, Margolis HS, Sheldon RE. Possible association between maternal indomethacin therapy and primary pulmonary hypertension of the newborn. Am J Obstet Gynecol 1976; 126:467–9.

[32] Eronen M, Pesonen E, Kurki T, et al. The effects of indomethacin and a β-sympathomimetic agent on the fetal ductus during treatment for preterm labor: a randomized double-blind study. Am J Obstet Gynecol 1991;164:141–6.

[33] Moise KJ. Effect of advancing gestational age on the frequency of fetal ductal constriction in the association with maternal indomethacin use. Am J Obstet Gynecol 1993;168:1350–3.

[34] Vermillion ST, Scardo JA, Lashus AG, et al. The effect of indomethacin tocolysis on fetal ductus arteriosus constriction with advancing gestational age. Am J Obstet Gynecol 1997;177:256–61.

[35] Moise KJ. Indomethacin therapy in the treatment of symptomatic polyhydramnios. Clin Obstet Gynecol 1991;34:310–8.

[36] Norton ME, Merrill J, Cooper BAB, et al. Neonatal complications after the administration of indomethacin for preterm labor. N Engl J Med 1993;329:1602–7.

[37] Vermillion ST, Newman RB. Recent indomethacin tocolysis is not associated with neonatal complication in preterm infants. Am J Obstet Gynecol 1999;181:1083–6.

[38] Ment LR, Duncan CC, Ehrenkranz RA, et al. Randomized low-dose indomethacin trial for prevention of intraventricular hemorrhage in very low birth weight neonates. J Pediatr 1988; 112:948–55.

[39] Souter D, Harding J, McCowan L, et al. Antenatal indomethacin: adverse fetal effects confirmed. Aust N Z J Obstet Gynaecol 1998;38:11–6.

[40] Pomeranz A, Korzets Z, Dolfin Z, et al. Acute renal failure in the neonate induced by the administration of indomethacin as a tocolytic agent. Nephrol Dial Transplant 1996;11:1139–41.

[41] Baerts W, Fetter WP, Hop WC, et al. Cerebral lesions in preterm infants after tocolytic indomethacin. Dev Med Child Neurol 1990;32:910–8.

[42] Mari G, Moise Jr KJ, Deter RL, et al. Doppler assessment of the pulsatility index of the middle cerebral artery during constriction of the fetal ductus arteriosus after indomethacin therapy. Am J Obstet Gynecol 1989;161(6 Pt 1):1528–31.

[43] Parilla BV, Tamura RK, Cohen LS, et al. Lack of effect of antenatal indomethacin on fetal cerebral blood flow. Am J Obstet Gynecol 1997;176:1166–9 [discussion: 1169–71].

[44] Major CA, Lewis DF, Harding JA, et al. Tocolysis with indomethacin increases the incidence of necrotizing enterocolitis in the low-birth-weight neonate. Am J Obstet Gynecol 1994;170: 102–6.

[45] Hanif R, Pittas A, Feng Y, et al. Effects of nonsteroidal anti-inflammatory drugs on proliferation and on induction of apoptosis in colon cancer cells by a prostaglandin-independent pathway. Biochem Pharmacol 1996;52:237–45.

[46] Slater D, Dennes W, Sawdy R, et al. Expression of cyclo-oxygenase types -1 and -2 in human fetal membranes throughout pregnancy. J Mol Endocrinol 1999;22:125–30.

[47] Olson DM, Mijovic JE, Zaragoza DB, et al. Prostaglandin endoperoxide H synthase type 1 and type 2 messenger ribonucleic acid in human fetal tissues throughout gestation and in the newborn infant. Am J Obstet Gynecol 2001;184:169–74.

[48] Hawkey CJ. Cox-2 inhibitors. Lancet 1999;353:307–14.

[49] Takahashi Y, Roman C, Chemtob S, et al. Cyclooxygenase-2 inhibitors constrict the fetal lamb ductus arteriosus both in vitro and in vivo. Am J Physiol Regul Integr Comp Physiol 2000; 278:R1496–505.

[50] Weeks JW, Mailhes JB, Lewis DF. Antenatal indomethacin exposure and neonatal intraventricular hemorrhage: a side effect or an association? Am J Obstet Gynecol 1997;176:1122–3.

[51] Gomez R, Ghezzi F, Romero R, et al. Premature labor and intra-amniotic infection: clinical aspects and role of the cytokines in diagnosis and pathophysiology. Clin Perinatol 1995;22: 281–342.

[52] Carlson SE, Montalto MB, Ponder DL, et al. Lower incidence of necrotizing enterocolitis in infants fed a preterm formula with egg phospholipids. Pediatr Res 1998;44:491–8.

[53] Komhoff M, Wang JL, Cheng HF, et al. Cyclooxygenase-2-selective inhibitors impair glomerulogenesis and renal cortical development. Kidney Int 2000;57:414–22.

[54] Peruzzi L, Gianoglio B, Porcellini MG, et al. Neonatal end-stage renal failure associated with maternal ingestion of cyclo-oxygenase-type-2 selective inhibitor. Lancet 1999;354:1615.

[55] Landau D, Shelef I, Polacheck H, et al. Perinatal vasoconstrictive renal insufficiency associated with maternal nimesulide use. Am J Perinatol 1999;16:441–4.

[56] Cantor B, Tyler T, Nelson RM, et al. Oligohydramnios and transient neonatal anuria: a possible association with the maternal use of prostaglandin synthetase inhibitors. J Reprod Med 1980;24: 220–3.

[57] Rac V, Lye S. Tocolysis due to the COX-2 inhibitor, meloxicam, is not associated with reduced expression of COX-2 and COX-1 protein in fetal kidney, lung, small intestine, adrenal gland, heart, liver, and brain of sheep preterm labor. Am J Obstet Gynecol 2003;189:S166.

[58] Sitka CS, Gross GA, Leguizamon G, et al. A prospective randomized safety trial of celecoxib for treatment of preterm labor. Am J Obstet Gynecol 2002;187:653–60.

[59] Slatterly MM, Friel AM, Healy DG, et al. Uterine relaxent effects of cyclooxygenase-2 inhibitors in vitro. Obstet Gynecol 2001;98:563–9.

[60] McWhorter J, Carlan SJ, O'Leary TD, et al. Rofecoxib versus magnesium sulfate to arrest preterm labor: a randomized trial. Obstet Gynecol 2004;103:923–30.

ELSEVIER
SAUNDERS

Obstet Gynecol Clin N Am
32 (2005) 519–525

OBSTETRICS AND
GYNECOLOGY
CLINICS
OF NORTH AMERICA

Use of Calcium Channel Antagonists for Preterm Labor

Adrienne Z. Ables, PharmD[a], Ana Maria Romero, MD[a],
Suneet P. Chauhan, MD[b],*

[a]Spartanburg Family Medicine Residency Program, 853 North Church Street, Suite 510,
Spartanburg, SC 29303, USA
[b]Department of Medical Education and Maternal-Fetal Medicine,
Spartanburg Regional Medical Center, 101 East Wood Street, Spartanburg, SC 29303, USA

Preterm birth is defined as delivery occurring before 37 weeks of gestation. The estimated incidence in the United States is 12% of all live births [1]. Risk factors associated with preterm labor are previous preterm birth, pregnancy body mass index less than 20, cigarette smoking, African American race, multiple pregnancy, bleeding in the second trimester, interpregnancy interval of less than 6 months, bacterial vaginosis at less than 16 weeks gestation, periodontal infection, gestational diabetes, and psychiatric disorders [2–8]. Preterm delivery is the leading cause of infant morbidity and mortality in developed countries, accounting for 75% of perinatal deaths [9]. Long-term sequelae include cerebral palsy, visual or hearing impairment, developmental delay, and chronic lung disease [10]. Preterm birth is a serious and costly health care problem accounting for approximately 35% of all United States health care spending for infants [11].

Many tocolytic drugs have been used to inhibit preterm labor including magnesium sulfate; β-mimetic agents; prostaglandin synthetase inhibitors (ie, indomethacin); and calcium channel antagonists (CCAs). This article focuses on the effectiveness and safety of CCAs as a therapeutic option in the management of preterm labor. Their first use was reported in 1972 by Mosler and Rosenboom [12]. Although they are considered a first-line treatment in Europe, CCAs remain as a second line of treatment in the United States [13,14].

---

* Corresponding author.
E-mail address: schauhan@srhs.com (S.P. Chauhan).

0889-8545/05/$ – see front matter © 2005 Elsevier Inc. All rights reserved.
doi:10.1016/j.ogc.2005.04.004   *obgyn.theclinics.com*

Goals of treatment

A short-term goal of the use of tocolytics is labor inhibition for at least 24 to 48 hours to administer glucocorticoids, which significantly decreases the incidence of respiratory distress syndrome, necrotizing enterocolitis, and severe intraventricular hemorrhage in newborns between 24 and 34 weeks of gestation [15]. Another short-term goal of prolonging pregnancy is to allow time for transfer to a tertiary care facility where a higher level of neonatal care is available. The use of tocolytics prolongs pregnancy sufficiently to reduce neonatal mortality and morbidity [16].

Mechanism of action

CCAs are potent uterine relaxants. They work by blocking voltage-dependent L-type calcium channels in cardiac muscle and vascular and nonvascular smooth muscle, including myometrial cells. In the pregnant uterus, they decrease the influx intracellular calcium ions and promote relaxation [17]. The dihydropyridine CCAs have less effect on the cardiac conduction system than older drugs like verapamil or diltiazem and are preferred for tocolysis. Nifedipine is the most widely studied CCA in the management of preterm labor.

Effectiveness

Nifedipine has been compared with ritodrine in an open randomized multi-center study [18]. The investigators followed 185 pregnant women diagnosed with preterm labor who received either oral nifedipine or intravenous ritodrine. They found that nifedipine postponed delivery longer than ritodrine and was associated with a significantly higher mean gestational age at birth and a higher mean birth weight. The higher tocolytic efficacy was associated with a lower incidence of neonatal morbidity related to respiratory distress syndrome (21% versus 37%); intracranial bleeding (18% versus 31%); and neonatal jaundice (52% versus 67%). Maternal side effects, such as nausea, vomiting, tachycardia, and anxiety, were severe and caused discontinuation in 13% of women treated with ritodrine. Nifedipine was not discontinued in any subject because of side effects.

Oral nifedipine was compared with magnesium sulfate in a randomized, controlled trial [19]. The researchers included 80 women who were in preterm labor at 20 to 34 weeks' gestation. There was no difference in tocolytic efficacy and neonatal mortality between the two groups. None of the nifedipine-treated women discontinued therapy, whereas 10% of magnesium-treated patients stopped treatment because of pulmonary edema or chest pain. The study authors concluded that oral nifedipine was as efficacious as intravenous magnesium sulfate but better tolerated.

Because of the relatively small sample sizes in the aforementioned studies, King and colleagues [20] conducted a systematic review of 12 randomized control trials including 1029 women in preterm labor. The trials compared CCAs with other tocolytic agents, mainly β-mimetics. CCAs significantly reduced the number of women giving birth within 7 days of receiving treatment and before 34 weeks of gestation (number needed to treat = 11). The use of CCAs was associated with a statistically significant increase in gestation at birth and a reduction in neonatal respiratory distress syndrome (RR, 0.63; 95% CI, 0.46–0.88); necrotizing enterocolitis (RR, 0.21; 95% CI, 0.05–0.96); intraventricular hemorrhage (RR, 0.59; 95% CI, 0.36–0.98); and neonatal jaundice (RR, 0.73; 95% CI, 0.57–0.93). Women who received CCAs were less likely to discontinue treatment because of adverse drug reactions when compared with other tocolytic agents. The number needed to treat for maternal adverse drug reaction requiring cessation of treatment was 14 and for any side effect it was 3. The authors concluded that CCAs are more effective tocolytic agents than other drugs and are better tolerated.

Side effects

Nifedipine is generally well tolerated in women with preterm labor. Documented maternal side effects include dizziness, lightheadedness, headache, flushing, nausea, and transient hypotension [21]. The side effects of various tocolytic regimens are compared in Table 1. Nifedipine-induced hypotension typically responds to positioning the mother in a left lateral recumbent position and elevating her feet. The combination of magnesium sulfate and nifedipine should be avoided because of case reports of symptomatic hypocalcemia, neuromuscular blockade, and cardiac toxicity, including maternal death [22–24]. In addition, there is a case report of a myocardial infarction in a 29-year-old woman who received nifedipine immediately after intravenous ritodrine therapy [25]. The patient and fetus survived without complications.

Animal studies have demonstrated a decrease in uteroplacental blood flow secondary to maternal hypotension induced by nicardipine infusion [26,27]. Human studies, however, have not supported significant changes in blood flow during tocolysis with oral nifedipine [28]. Most importantly, CCAs have not been shown adversely to affect the fetus [29,30]. There was no significant increase in congenital anomalies among 586 mothers who had been exposed to CCAs as compared with 907 controls (2.6% versus 2.4%, respectively) [31].

Contraindications

The only true contraindication to the use of nifedipine is hypersensitivity to the drug. Women with established coronary artery disease or cerebrovascular disease also are not candidates for nifedipine treatment because hypotensive

Table 1
Side effects of tocolytic therapy

Tocolytic agent	Maternal side effects	Fetal side effects
Betamimetics	Arrhythmia Pulmonary edema Myocardial ischemia Tachycardia Shortness of breath Hypotension Hyperglycemia Hypokalemia Tremor Nervousness Nausea or vomiting	Tachycardia Hyperinsulinemia Fetal hyperglycemia Neonatal hypoglycemia Hypocalcemia Hypotension Ileus
Calcium channel blockers	Transient hypotension Headache Flushing Dizziness Nausea Palpitations	None known
Prostaglandin inhibitors	Gastritis, nausea Proctitis with hematochezia Impairment of renal function Increased postpartum hemorrhage	Oligohydramnios Constriction of ductus arteriosus Necrotizing enterocolitis Intraventricular hemorrhage
Magnesium sulfate	Flushing Nausea and vomiting Diplopia, blurred vision Headache Lethargy Ileus Hypocalcemia Muscle weakness Pulmonary edema Cardiac arrest	Hypotonia, lethargy Bone demineralization

Data from: Refs. [32–47].

episodes could theoretically lead to myocardial infarction or stroke. Fortunately these chronic illnesses are infrequently encountered in the obstetric population.

Dosing and administration

After ingestion, nifedipine has an onset of action of about 20 minutes and peak plasma concentrations are reached at 30 to 60 minutes. Elimination half-life is 2 to 3 hours. Nifedipine is available as an immediate release formulation in 10- and 20-mg capsules and 30-, 60-, and 90-mg extended-release tablets. The dose of nifedipine for the management of preterm labor varies across clinical

Table 2
Costs of tocolytic agents

Tocolytic regimen	Cost[a]
Calcium channel blockers: nifedipine	
Loading dose: 30 mg po	$1.84–2.68
Maintenance dose: 10–20 mg po every 4–6 h	$1.84–5.46/d
Betamimetic: terbutaline	
0.25 mg subcutaneously every 20 min to 3 h (hold for pulse >120 beats per min)	$32.49 per course
Magnesium sulfate:	
IV tubing	$2.86
Loading dose: 4–6 g IV over 20 min	$1.36–1.86
Maintenance dose: 2–3 g IV per h	$16.32/d (drug without fluid or preparation costs) $26.01/d (premixed bags)
Prostaglandin synthetase inhibitors: indomethacin	
Loading dose: 50 mg pr or 50–100 mg po	$0.65–1.30
Maintenance dose: 25–50 mg po every 6 h × 48 h	$1.79–3.96 per day course

[a] Costs calculated using Average Wholesale Price (Drug Topics Red Book: Montvale, NJ; 2004).

trials; however, a typical regimen consists of a loading dose of 10 mg by mouth every 20 to 30 minutes if contractions persist, up to 40 mg within the first hour [32]. A maintenance dose of 10 to 20 mg every 4 to 6 hours is recommended. Extended-release nifedipine may also be used at a daily dose of 60 to 160 mg. Duration of treatment has yet to be established. The costs of various tocolytic drug regimens are summarized in Table 2.

Summary

As the rate of preterm delivery rises, it is becoming increasingly clear that the major role of tocolytics is prolongation of pregnancy to optimize the benefit of corticosteroids and, if necessary, permit transfer to a tertiary center. Based on effectiveness, there is no first-line tocolytic agent but considering the cost, ease of administration, and lower likelihood of side effects, nifedipine should be used more often and perhaps even replace magnesium sulfate.

References

[1] Martin JA, Hamilton BE, Ventura SJ, et al. Births: final data for 2001. Natl Vital Stat Rep 2002;51:1–104.
[2] Iams JD. Preterm birth. In: Gabbe SG, Niebyl JR, Simpson JL, editors. Obstetrics: normal and problem pregnancies. 4th edition. New York: Churchill Livingstone; 2002. p. 775–826.

[3] Leitich H, Bodner-Adler B, Brunbauer M, et al. Bacterial vaginosis as a risk factor for preterm delivery: a meta-analysis. Am J Obstet Gynecol 2003;189:139–47.

[4] Jeffcoat MK, Geurs NC, Reddy MS, et al. Periodontal infection and preterm birth: results of prospective study. J Am Dent Assoc 2001;132:875–80.

[5] Moutquin JM. Socio-economic and psychosocial factors in the management and prevention of preterm labor. Br J Obstet Gynaecol 2003;110:56–60.

[6] Smith GC, Pell JP, Dobbie R. Interpregnancy interval and risk of preterm birth and neonatal death: retrospective cohort study. BMJ 2003;327:313–9.

[7] Kelly RH, Russo J, Holt VL, et al. Psychiatric and substance use disorders as risk factors for low birth weight and preterm delivery. Obstet Gynecol 2002;100:297–304.

[8] Hedderson MM, Ferrara A, Sacks DA. Gestational diabetes mellitus and lesser degrees of pregnancy hyperglycemia: association with increased risk of spontaneous preterm birth. Obstet Gynecol 2003;102:850–6.

[9] Demissie K, Rhoads GG, Ananth CV, et al. Trends in preterm birth and neonatal mortality among blacks and whites in the United States from 1989 to 1997. Am J Epidemiol 2001; 154:307–15.

[10] Hack M, Taylor HG, Klein N, et al. School-age outcomes in children with birth weight under 750 g. N Engl J Med 1994;331:753–9.

[11] Lewit EM, Baker LS, Corman H, et al. The direct cost of low birth weight. Future Child 1995;5:35–56.

[12] Mosler KH, Rosenboom HG. Newer possibilities of tocolytic treatment in obstetrics. Z Geburtshilfe Perinatol 1972;176:85–96.

[13] Norwitz ER, Robinson JN, Challis JRG. The control of labor. N Engl J Med 1999;341:660–6.

[14] Bennett P, Edwards D. Use of magnesium sulphate in obstetrics. Lancet 1997;350:1491.

[15] Crowley P. Prophylactic corticosteroids for preterm birth (Cochrane Review). In: The Cochrane Library, Issue 4. Oxford: Update Software; 2003.

[16] Slattery MM, Morrison JJ. Preterm delivery. Lancet 2002;360:1489–97.

[17] McDonald TF, Pelzer S, Trautwein W, et al. Regulation and modulation of calcium channels in cardiac, skeletal, and smooth muscle cells. Physiol Rev 1994;74:365–507.

[18] Papatsonis DNM, Kok JH, Van Geijn HP, et al. Neonatal effects of nifedipine and ritodrine for preterm labor. Obstet Gynecol 2000;95:477–81.

[19] Glock JL, Morales WJ. Efficacy and safety of nifedipine versus magnesium sulfate in the management of preterm labor: a randomized study. Am J Obstet Gynecol 1993;169:960–4.

[20] King JF, Flenady BJ, Papatsonis DNM, et al. Calcium channel blockers for inhibiting preterm labour (Cochrane Review). In: The Cochrane Library, Issue 3. Oxford: Update Software; 2003.

[21] Hearne AE, Nagey DA. Therapeutic agents in preterm labor: tocolytic agents. Clin Obstet Gynecol 2000;43:787–801.

[22] Koontz SL, Friedman SA, Schwartz ML. Symptomatic hypocalcemia after tocolytic therapy with magnesium sulfate and nifedipine. Am J Obstet Gynecol 2004;190:1773–6.

[23] Snyder SW, Cardwell MS. Neuromuscular blockade with magnesium sulfate and nifedipine. Am J Obstet Gynecol 1989;161:35–6.

[24] Davis WB, Wells SR, Kuller JA, et al. Analysis of the risks associated with calcium channel blockade: implications for the obstetrician-gynecologist. Obstet Gynecol Surv 1997;52: 198–201.

[25] Oei SG, Oei SK, Brolmann HAM. Myocardial infarction during nifedipine therapy for preterm labor. N Engl J Med 1999;340:154.

[26] Parisi VM, Salinas J, Stockmar EJ. Fetal vascular responses to maternal nicardipine administration in the hypertensive ewe. Am J Obstet Gynecol 1989;161:1035–9.

[27] Lirette M, Holbrook RH, Katz M. Cardiovascular and uterine blood flow changes during nicardipine HCl tocolysis in the rabbit. Obstet Gynecol 1987;69:79–82.

[28] Mari G, Kirshon B, Moise Jr KJ, et al. Doppler assessment of the fetal and uroplacental circulation during nifedipine therapy for preterm labor. Am J Obstet Gynecol 1989;161:1514–8.

[29] Sorensen HT, Steffensen FH, Olesen C, et al. Pregnancy outcome in women exposed to calcium channel blockers. Reprod Toxicol 1998;12:383–4.

[30] Magee LA, Schick B, Donnefeld AE, et al. The safety of calcium channel blockers in human pregnancy: a prospective, multicenter cohort study. Am J Obstet Gynecol 1996;174:823–8.

[31] Sorensen HT, Czeizel AE, Rockenbauer M, et al. The risk of limb deficiencies and other congenital abnormalities in children exposed in utero to calcium channel blockers. Acta Obstet Gynecol Scand 2001;80:397–401.

[32] American College of Obstetricians and Gynecologists. Management of preterm labor. ACOG practical bulletin No. 43. Washington: ACOG; 2003.

[33] Gordon M, Samuels P. Indomethacin. Clin Obstet Gynecol 1995;38:697–705.

[34] Steiger RM, Boyd EL, Powers DR, et al. Acute maternal renal insufficiency in premature labor treated with indomethacin. Am J Perinatol 1993;10:381–3.

[35] Panter KR, Mannah ME, Amankwah KS, et al. The effect of indomethacin tocolysis in preterm labor on perinatal outcome: a randomized placebo-controlled trial. Br J Obstet Gynecol 1999; 106:467–73.

[36] de Wit W, van Mourik I, Wiesenhaan PF. Prolonged maternal indomethacin therapy associated with oligohydramnios. Br J Obstet Gynaecol 1988;95:303–5.

[37] Hendricks SK, Smith JR, Moore DE, et al. Oligohydramnios associated with prostaglandin synthetase inhibitors in preterm labor. Br J Obstet Gynaecol 1990;97:312–6.

[38] Niebyl JR, Witter FR. Neonatal outcome after indomethacin treatment for preterm labor. Am J Obstet Gynecol 1986;155:747–9.

[39] Norton M, Merill J, Cooper B, et al. Neonatal complications after the administration of indomethacin for preterm labor. N Engl J Med 1993;329:1602–7.

[40] Major CA, Lewis DF, Harding JA, et al. Tocolysis with indomethacin increases the incidence of necrotizing enterocolitis in the low-birth-weight neonate. Am J Obstet Gynecol 1994;170: 102–6.

[41] Tsatsaris V, Papatsonis D, Goffinet F, et al. Tocolysis with nifedipine or beta-adrenergic agonists: a meta-analysis. Obstet Gynecol 2001;97:840–7.

[42] Leveno KJ, Cunningham FG. Beta-adrenergic agonists for preterm labor. N Engl J Med 1992;327:349–51.

[43] Young DC, Toofanian A, Leveno KJ. Potassium and glucose concentrations without treatment during ritodrine tocolysis. Am J Obstet Gynecol 1983;145:105–6.

[44] Brazy JE, Pupkin MJ. Effects of maternal isoxsuprine administration on preterm infants. J Pediatr 1979;94:444–8.

[45] Green KW, Key TC, Coen R, et al. The effects of maternally administered magnesium sulfate on the neonate. Am J Obstet Gynecol 1983;81:185–8.

[46] Holcomb WL, Shackelford GD, Petrie RH. Magnesium tocolysis and neonatal bone abnormalities: a controlled study. Obstet Gynecol 1991;78:611–4.

[47] Hearne AE, Nagey DA. Therapeutic agents in preterm labor: tocolytic agents. Clin Obstet Gynecol 2000;43:787–801.

ELSEVIER
SAUNDERS

Obstet Gynecol Clin N Am
32 (2005) 527–532

OBSTETRICS AND
GYNECOLOGY
CLINICS
OF NORTH AMERICA

Index

Note: Page numbers of article titles are in **boldface** type.

A

Activin, as marker, for preterm labor, 378

β-Agonists, for preterm labor, **457–484**
  choice of, 462
  contraindications to, 478
  efficacy of, 460–462
  FDA approved, 458–459
  fetal and neonatal effects of, 464
  in twin and multiple gestations,
    435–436
  maternal effects of, 462–463
  physiology of, 459–460
  protocol for, 464–465,
    477–478, 479
  side effects of, 461
  subcutaneous pump administration
    of, 465–479
    costs of, 476, 478–479
    efficacy of, 468–471
    in multiple gestations,
      469–470
    safety of, 476
  versus magnesium sulfate,
    492–493

Alpha-fetoprotein, as marker, for preterm labor,
  377–378

Alvarez waves, assessment of, 342, 345–346

Amniotic fluid culture, for intrauterine
  infections, in preterm labor, 398

Amniotic fluid volume, measurement of, for
  oligohydramnios, 509

Amoxicillin, for preterm premature rupture
  of membranes, remote from term (before
  32 weeks), 421–422

Ampicillin, for preterm premature rupture
  of membranes, remote from term (before
  32 weeks), 421

Antibiotics, for intrauterine infections,
  399–402
  for preterm premature rupture of
    membranes, 420

remote from term (before
  32 weeks), 420–422
with cerclage, for cervical incompetence,
  449–450, 452

Antiprostaglandin drugs, for preterm labor,
  501–517
  cyclooxygenase isotype expression
    by, 504
  cyclooxygenase specificity of,
    503–504
  efficacy of, 505–506, 513–514
  fetal and neonatal effects of,
    507–511
    prevention of, 508
    surveillance for, 508
  mechanism of action of, 501–503
  pharmacokinetics of, 504–505
  rationale for, 511–512
  safety of, 512–513, 514
  versus magnesium sulfate, 491
  with magnesium sulfate, 494

B

Bacterial vaginosis, and preterm birth,
  403–404

Bacteriuria, and intrauterine infections, 402

Biochemical markers, for preterm labor,
  369–381
  activin, 378
  alpha-fetoprotein, 377–378
  corticotropin-releasing hormone,
    375–377
  estriol, 373–375
    salivary samples of, 374–375
    versus modified Creasy score,
      374–375
  fetal fibronectin, 370–373
    Tli testing system for, 373
  β-human chorionic gonadotropin,
    377–378
  inhibin, 378
  relaxin, 378

ELSEVIER
SAUNDERS

Obstet Gynecol Clin N Am
32 (2005) 527–532

OBSTETRICS AND
GYNECOLOGY
CLINICS
OF NORTH AMERICA

Index

Note: Page numbers of article titles are in **boldface** type.

0889-8545/05/$ – see front matter © 2005 Elsevier Inc. All rights reserved.
doi:10.1016/S0889-8545(05)00047-1
obgyn.theclinics.com

Changing Your Address?

Make sure your subscription changes too! When you notify us of your new address, you can help make our job easier by including an exact copy of your Clinics label number with your old address (see illustration below.) This number identifies you to our computer system and will speed the processing of your address change. Please be sure this label number accompanies your old address and your corrected address—you can send an old Clinics label with your number on it or just copy it exactly and send it to the address listed below.

We appreciate your help in our attempt to give you continuous coverage. Thank you.

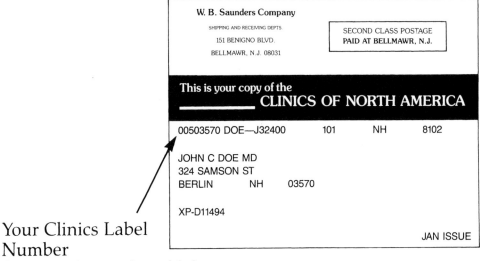

Your Clinics Label Number
Copy it exactly or send your label along with your address to:
W.B. Saunders Company, Customer Service
Orlando, FL 32887-4800
Call Toll Free 1-800-654-2452

Please allow four to six weeks for delivery of new subscriptions and for processing address changes.